Praise for
Own Your Wellness

"DANIELLA WRITES HER OWN authentic voice, presenting a compelling collection of ideas to improve your health and well-being, but most importantly, she's focused on helping you discover the way that's best for you!"

—*David,* CLIENT OF TEN YEARS

"*OWN YOUR WELLNESS* is a great addition to any health and wellness library. Daniella has done a wonderful job of collecting information, organizing it into well-thought-out sections, and explaining everything scientifically but clearly. If you want to start taking your health, fitness, and wellness into your own hands, don't hesitate to buy this book and read it from cover to cover; you'll be on your way to a healthier lifestyle in no time!"

—*Kim Rappaport, MD*

"DANIELLA HAS WORKED with me to dial in a unique wellness plan for my very rare and challenging health condition (Late Onset Tay Sachs). She helped me find an exercise, diet, and supplement regimen that best suits me and my goals, and this book will provide the same for you."

—*Vera Pesotchinsky,* CLIENT OF EIGHTEEN YEARS

"I HIGHLY RECOMMEND reading *Own Your Wellness*. The insights and guidance Daniella has given me over the thirteen years I have known and worked with her have helped me physically and mentally, even with the challenges of arthrogryposis. A must-read book for anyone wanting a book to help them help themselves."

—*Lisa Blanchette*

"IF YOU WANT TO take ownership of your wellness, this book is required reading. Daniella Dayoub Forrest has written the playbook for constructing a tailored and actionable plan to take your health to the next level. Insightful, practical, and very direct, Own Your Wellness will keep you honest on this important journey."

—*Donna Weber,* CONSULTANT AND AUTHOR OF
ONBOARDING MATTERS, HOW TO TURN
NEW CUSTOMERS INTO LOYAL CHAMPIONS

Own Your Wellness

Giving You the Tools to Break Through Your Health Plateaus

Daniella Dayoub Forrest

Forefront
BOOKS

Published by Forefront Books, Nashville, Tennessee.
Distributed by Simon & Schuster.

Library of Congress Control Number: 2023924647

Print ISBN: 978-1-63763-287-1
E-book ISBN: 978-1-63763-288-8

Cover Design by Michelle Manley, Graphique Design Co.
Interior Design by Mary Susan Oleson, Blu Design Concepts

Printed in the United States of America

To my grandparents, JJ and Darlene—
Thank you for teaching me that health
and happiness come from within,
that words matter, and that getting
lost in a book is the best place to be.
I'm grateful that my book will
take its place in your discerning library.

Contents

Foreword

I n the ever-evolving landscape of health and wellness, where
trends rise and fall and quick fixes are becoming the norm,
it is a great honor to introduce a book that resonates with the
wisdom and experience of a high-end health coach who firmly
roots herself in the real world. This book, written by my wife,
personal trainer, and built-in health coach, Daniella Dayoub
Forrest, stands as a testament to her compassion, insight, and
ability to put that in play.

Daniella is an extraordinary individual who has
constantly confronted the human condition with unyielding
honesty. Her unique journey as a health coach in the heart of
Silicon Valley has provided her with a distinct vantage point.
In this epicenter of innovation and entrepreneurship, where
her clients are at the cutting edge of technology, and the latest
theories, Daniella has undertaken the role of a discerning
critic. She's scrutinized a myriad of health trends, analyzing
them on their merit, never blindly embracing the newest fad.
What makes her unique is she isn't rigid in her own philosophy but integrates new information into a personalized
approach for each of her clients.

Born to a mother who held the title of Miss Texas in
1975, Daniella inherited a legacy of grace and poise. Yet,
her mother's influence goes far beyond beauty pageants;
she passed down a genius-level intellect and wicked deter-
mination. Growing up in a household that valued both her
father's relentless work ethic as a successful business owner in
El Paso, Texas, and her mother's grace, she developed a deep

appreciation for the value of hard work and discipline. In a family where appearance was an undeniable priority, it sent her on a path of health and fitness.

Daniella's journey led her to navigate the labyrinth of trendy diets, explore the terrain of fad workouts, and grapple with her own battles concerning eating habits. Emerging from these experiences, she garnered an intimate understanding of what it genuinely takes to progress in health and wellness. Her humility and candidness about her own journey make her as real as it gets in a world often obscured by unrealistic ideals and shallow solutions.

At the core of Daniella's philosophy lies a profound belief that the human body is an adaptable machine. Her guiding principle is both simple and profound: when you encounter an impasse, be prepared to adapt and adjust as necessary. Whether it be tweaks to diet, exercise, or supplements, this foundational insight underscores her approach. This principle allows her to help her clients see results and stay on target before losing faith.

What truly distinguishes Daniella is her extraordinary combination of hyperintelligence and next-level EQ, allowing her to hyper-focus on her clients' words and emotions. Then, with remarkable finesse, she deciphers complex issues and distills them into simple, actionable steps.

She takes the vast library of her mind and translates it into a language her clients can understand, relate to, and act upon.

This book serves as a twenty-year cheat code, unlocking the intricate workings of Daniella's remarkable mind and the profound influence she has had on the lives of her clients. It provides an open window into her world of transformation, where she empowers individuals to rekindle their lost vitality, break free from the bonds of stagnation, and reach levels of well-being they may never have thought possible.

As I delved into this book for the first time, I couldn't help but be astounded by its precise representation of Daniella's approach, which has inspired and actively guided countless individuals over the years. Her words are not mere lessons; they are nuggets of simple genius. These nuggets, given to her clients when they are stuck and struggling, help them get to where they want to be.

What truly sets this book apart is that it doesn't impose upon you the need to unquestioningly adopt the latest trend. Instead of urging you to make a slew of changes that often lead to confusion, Daniella's approach is about helping you discover what works best for you. *Own Your Wellness* is designed to assist you, regardless of whether you are low-carb, paleo, vegetarian, or a carnivore. This book will guide you to the next level with your existing lifestyle or program by helping you fine-tune your plan. In a world where health advice frequently follows a one-size-fits-all approach, this book is a breath of fresh air, offering a personalized path that meets you where you are and empowers you to grow from there.

As you dig into the pages of this book, I hope that you approach it with a receptive mind. Daniella has gifted us with an extraordinary blueprint for living a better life. Her insights, experiences, and dedication to enhancing the lives of others shine through every page. May this book become your trusted guide, a loyal companion, and an enduring source of inspiration as you chart your unique path to a healthier, happier, and more vibrant you.

Gregg Forrest

INTRODUCTION

Owning Your Wellness

"Owning your wellness" is essential to any health journey. It means that you are in charge of your body, your health, your state of mind—your wellness. Over all the years I've been coaching people, one theme comes up again and again … and again—people just want me to tell them what to do. They want me to hold them accountable, and they want tangible results. I can't tell you the number of times I've had people say to me, "Just tell me what to eat and when, and I'll do it." But if I did that, I would be the one in charge of their wellness. Not them. I would be at the helm of their decision-making, and I'd be responsible for their success even. It took me a few years to understand why people wanted me to be in charge, why they wanted me to "just tell them what to do!" The real reason was that, ultimately, they didn't want to be responsible if they failed. They wanted to be able to blame their lack of weight loss, lack of energy, lack of muscle tone, or just general "lack" on me!

Once I figured that out, I was not going to fall for it anymore—no more telling people precisely what to eat and at what time. I was no longer going to give them any promises of weight loss, increased energy, or muscle tone. Nope. It was time to shift my teaching and encouragement to all my clients to finally own their wellness! As a health coach, it's my job to educate, encourage, question, guide, sometimes console, and often celebrate. But it is not my responsibility

> Owning your wellness is ultimately up to you.

15

if someone doesn't reach their goals. Owning your wellness is ultimately up to you. It's your body, your life, and your future. As your guide, I will help you uncover what is working and what is not. I will show you ways to reframe your thinking and regroup your efforts. I will help you make decisions to support your goals. I'll even massage those goals with you to make sure they are not just attainable but worthwhile. I'm here to help you "own your wellness!"

How to Use This Book

You don't need to go through this book cover to cover. You may find it helpful to skip among the chapters (Nourish, Move, Explore, Enhance, and Putting It All Together). If you go straight to the back, you will find a large workbook section. There I help you distill the information you find helpful into actionable items for you to move forward. In fact, you may find it best to take a look at the "Putting It All Together" chapter first to get an idea of what things to go back to and make notes on. Within the book, there are smaller areas to make notes on how the concepts would apply to your unique situation. From figuring out your goals and understanding your "why" to specifics on how to eat, move, test, and supplement, that whole workbook section is where you take those notes and map out your personal "Own Your Wellness" journey. All of the charts and notes are available for download at dfitlife.com/own-your-wellness-resources/.

Remember, the key to owning your wellness is putting ideas into the context of *you*.

Figuring Out Your "Why"

One of the most important things you can do to own your wellness is to figure out your "why." Why do you want to be fitter? Why do you want to eat healthier? Why do you want to get into those old skinny jeans? Why???

Your "why" matters more than you realize. Your "why" is the key to owning your wellness and, ultimately, the key to your success. Whenever I have seen clients struggle to achieve their goals or, worse, give up on them, it is often tied up in not having their "why" figured out. If you are working toward a goal for no reason, you are not likely to succeed!

Imagine you were putting money into your savings account with the ultimate goal of having $250,000. You sit down, look at your monthly income and expenses, and decide how much you will squirrel away monthly to reach that goal. Based on that assessment, it looks like it will take you about two and a half years. So, you're in for thirty months of putting away every extra penny. The first month goes great. You put a whopping $8,500 into your account (why not start out ahead?). The next month, you put in $8,000 (you know, you did overdo it last month). In the third month, you have your first post-pandemic tropical vacation planned and decide just to skip this month altogether. Of course, said vacation was a-ma-zing! So, it is probably best to pay off those credit cards instead of depositing money into that savings account. By month five, you've forgotten about the goal and are just going to keep that $16,500 in there for a rainy day. Missed it by thaaaat much!

Okay, so where did this go wrong? You had a plan, and it was attainable based on your analysis. Your only real mistake was that you had no "why"! What was the quarter million for? A down payment on a house? A rental property? A huge business investment? A serious goal requires a serious, intentional, and, most importantly, meaningful reason to attain it. You need a good "why."

When we apply this thinking to your wellness, your chances of success increase infinitely! If your goal is to lose ten pounds, we have to help you figure out why. Maybe it's because you have a major event coming up, and that killer outfit waiting in your closet fits only when you're down ten more pounds. Or maybe it's something more meaningful: maybe that ten pounds puts you at a healthy BMI (Body Mass Index: the ratio of your height to your weight), and therefore losing the weight and keeping it off might help you live longer. Or maybe your ten-pound weight loss is what you need to prove to yourself that you can lose the next fifty in order to achieve long-term health and be there for your loved ones. I don't know about you, but those last two sound like more meaningful reasons that will truly help keep you on track.

Obviously, wellness encompasses so many other things besides weight loss. I will spend a fair amount of time in this book talking about the myriad of ways you can own your wellness. Regardless of the category your personal goal fits into, it is critical that you find a "why" that really resonates, that sings to you, that makes you emotional, that motivates you, that you can refer to again and again and again when things get hard. You need a "why" that matters!

Often I find it best to ask "who?" in addition to "why?" Who will benefit from your success? Do you have a spouse, child, parent, or friend who needs you to be healthy? Maybe you have a dog or cat that depends on you being able to care for them. If you are in a romantic relationship, think about how your improved health can add to your partnership with that person. As a parent (or pet parent), how can you model healthy daily living? If you are caring for a parent, child, or whomever, how can being more fit and healthier help you provide them with better care? If you're struggling at work or want to strive for a better job, how can your wellness be a step in the right direction?

There's nothing wrong with wanting to lose a few pounds, clear up your skin, or put on some muscle for the mere idea of looking better in the mirror. But those goals will take you only so far. Yes, looking at yourself in the mirror and liking—no, loving—what you see is very much what I want for you and all of us. But when you can find a way to tie in increasing self-love and acceptance with a larger purpose, then you will be on the right track. *Imagine setting your sights on a wellness goal that makes you feel like the best possible version of yourself.* Imagine how great that version of you will interact with the world around you. You can do anything when your mind, body, and soul are lined up! You can be a rock star at work. You can be the parent you want to be for your children. You can support your parents as they did you. You can be there to hold your lover's hand through all life throws at you.

As I walk you through my methods and ways of thinking about wellness, keep these questions in mind. Remind yourself: "Why am I doing this?" "Why does this matter?" "How will this propel me to be that person I know is hiding within?"

Here are some questions you might consider in figuring out your "why":

How would being healthier and more energetic help me care for_____?	
If I felt better about my self-image, what other changes might that lead to?	
Besides myself, who in my life would benefit from seeing a healthier me?	
Insert your own question here.	

My "Why"

In writing this, I'm hopeful that I can provide you with all the ways I help my health coaching clients individually. Over the years, one of the hardest things for me has been finding a way to scale my business: to give many people the boost they need to own their wellness while maintaining my individualized attention. In fact, it's that one-on-one, unique-to-each-person coaching I give that is exactly why it's almost impossible for me to give generalized recommendations. Of course, you can easily go online and find advice on losing weight on a low-carb diet or doing HIIT (High-Intensity Interval Training) workouts to rev your metabolism. You can find all the coaching you want within minutes with the right search words. However, figuring out what works for *you* and only you is my "why."

Over the next several chapters, I will show you ways to nourish yourself, move daily, explore healing opportunities, and even play with enhancements. I will give you options and ideas to constantly evolve and progress. I'll help you figure out what works for you and what doesn't. You'll learn to assess when things need tweaking and when to pull back your efforts. Your wellness is unique and ever-changing. The diet and exercise routine you did in your twenties probably isn't going to cut it in your sixties. Just because your friend lost thirty pounds on the keto diet doesn't mean you will. Navigating all the advice online is a daunting task, and I'm here to help you. Together we'll parse through the information and show you strategies to apply it to your unique situation. I will help you put all the myriad pieces of health advice into the context of *you*.

When you can find ways to constantly evolve your efforts to help you consistently progress your health, then you are truly owning your wellness. If I just tell you what to do, and you execute, then I am the one owning it. I want you to find your own path, learn how to navigate the twists and turns, and continue to chart your own course. I believe that this is a huge missing link in what is wrong with the health and wellness industry right now. Although we have the tools to self-quantify and self-analyze, many people still want to be sheep. They want to be told what to do, how to do it, and be done. Unfortunately, that just doesn't work over the long term. You may be able to get results from a prescribed workout routine or diet regimen at first, but to stay fit and strong over the entirety of your lifespan, you're going to have to learn to be your own boss—to own your wellness!

It is so important to me that I empower people with the tools they need to be healthy for the rest of their lives that I base my success on client attrition. I want to say goodbye. I want my clients to feel like they have learned all they need to progress on their own and that they no longer need to work with me. It may sound crazy, but that is how I measure my coaching success. Nothing makes me happier than to hear a client say to me, "Daniella, this has been great. I have learned so much from you, and I feel amazing. I just don't think I need to keep having our sessions." When a client breaks up with me like that, my heart sings! Saying goodbye is my ultimate goal.

When you complete this book, I hope that you, too, will be able to say, "Goodbye and thank you, Daniella." I hope that you'll spend time filling out all the workbook sections to go back and reflect on them. I hope that you'll send a copy to anyone you know who is also struggling to own their wellness. I hope that you'll come back years from now and review what worked for you back then and how you can further evolve your efforts to fit the new you. The contents of this book are not time and space specific. While technologies and information will be new, the basic premises will be the same. You can always come back here, again and again, to touch up areas that need attention so that you never lose sight of owning your wellness.

The Only Constant Is Change

If there is one mantra, one phrase that I have leaned on and identified with my whole life, it is that "the only constant is change." When life seems too tumultuous for me to handle, I remind myself of this. When the future seems horribly uncertain, I go back to this. This is the only phrase that calms me when the world appears to be upside down and even moving backward. I'm not even sure why, really. It's not necessarily a comforting phrase. But somehow, reminding myself that we are always in flux, that things are always evolving, settles my mind. How can I be anxious about current chaos if things are always changing? What's the point in spinning out about the momentary craziness if it will soon be a distant memory? And before you roll your eyes too far into the back of your head and shut this book, please know that I am trying to be hyperbolic here. Constant change is at the root of my entire business and coaching model. You can't own your wellness without embracing this critical concept.

In fact, "constant change" is such a big part of me that it is represented in the only tattoo I have on my body! On

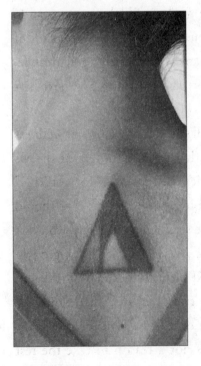

the back of my neck, you'll find the DFitLife logo (well, it was my tattoo long before I launched my business). When I decided to take my training business out on my own as an independent contractor back in 2007, I was racking my brain for ideas for my logo. My dear friend said to me, "Hey, you already have it, it's on your neck!" Duh. What else can better signify what I was trying to accomplish with my clients?

The delta (triangle) stands for "change" in an equation. And, of course, the K represents a constant. The colors represent the moods and feelings you have throughout the evolution. And, well, our lives/health/goals are always in a state of constant change ... thus ... the logo ...

Just because change and evolution are inevitable doesn't mean you are at the whim of wherever the wind blows you. This is where owning your wellness fits into the mix. Knowing that you are a dynamic creature in a dynamic world needs to be part of your strategy. As you are making changes and setting new goals, you should keep in mind where you have come from and where you are trying to go. The goal should not be to stay the same. The goal should be to constantly shift your methods to help you embrace the new version of yourself. How can you make small tweaks to your lifestyle, habits, and strategies to support the maturing and next-best version of you?

And please do not let small speed bumps in your wellness journey derail your efforts. If there is one thing that throws off my clients time and again, it's the idea of "all or nothing." Your wellness journey is not going to be perfect. Nor should it be. If it were so easy as to be seamless, you likely wouldn't have to pick up this darn book. When you are driving down the street and come to a speed bump, do you stop the car, get out, and give up on your trip? Uh, no! That would be ridiculous. Having a meal that doesn't fit in with your goals, or missing a day of exercise, is not a reason to take the rest of the day, week, or month off. You don't have to tank your efforts for now and just start over again later when it feels like it will be more convenient. You go over the speed bump and then resume the journey. **Don't use the speed bump as an excuse for taking a break. It is the break.** Those speed bumps/digressions/cheat meals/and so on are what will keep you sane over the long haul of your wellness journey. Keep your eyes on the road and remember where you are headed.

Aspects of Owning Your Wellness

What will you be focusing your efforts on as you travel the path to owning your wellness? Once you know why you are reaching for your goal, you have to figure out how, and that is what I'm here for. I will show you some exciting ways to work on getting healthier as you "own your wellness." To do this, I break up the various aspects of health into four categories:

Nourish

Move

Explore

Enhance

Nourish: When I coach people regarding diet, I don't just focus on food. What are you taking in? How are you taking it in? And, of course, why are you taking it in?

Move: Again, instead of zeroing in on "exercise" per se, I like to coach my clients to just move. That can be a lot of things, but as long as you are honoring your basic human need for movement, that's all that matters.

Explore: Here's where we dig deeper into the intricacies of how your body is working. Do you need to do some self-quantifying? Maybe it's time to look at some testing in relation to hormone function, detoxification, gut function, food sensitivities, and so on.

Enhance: I put this one last because adding in things like supplements should be icing on the delicious cake of your health. This is where we fill in some blanks with strategic supplements.

So let's dig in and start this journey together.

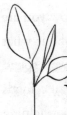

CHAPTER ONE

Nourish

I prefer to use the word "nourish" over "nutrition" because it encapsulates all that it means to feed yourself. When we focus on nourishing your health, it changes the conversation from just getting your fruits and veggies to how you are supporting your long-term health. It is not just about what you're eating, but how, when, and why. Of course, we'll spend some time here talking about how to choose specific foods and diet plans, but all of that is set in the context of helping your decision-making skills over the rest of your lifespan. I want you to own your wellness when it comes to nourishing yourself today, and for many decades to come.

Eat to Support Your Goals

Sadly, this idea is not discussed very much in the current dogma of nutrition. I feel like every time I get online, all I see are articles and blogs about how to "do keto right," or how to avoid added sugars and salt, or what the perfect fasting window is. If you've been taking notes and paying attention to what you've already read, you know exactly what is wrong with all of those articles: they lack *your "why"*!

First, we have to figure out what your goals are. Then we can make decisions to help you support them. If your goal is to maintain lean muscle mass and not lose or gain any more weight, then you should be making very different decisions than someone who needs to lose fifty pounds or gain fifteen. Your "why" will be quite different too. Maybe your goal is to keep your autoimmune condition from flaring up. Why? Because then you are not in pain, and you have a better quality of life. Once we know what and why, making decisions around that situation becomes so much clearer!

At the very end of this chapter, I will give you several different scenarios that might be related to your particular why and what. But before we get to specifics, I'd like to spend some time speaking in rather generalized terms. Most of what you will read over the next several pages will be geared toward the average adult aiming to optimize their body composition, energy, and mental acuity. But don't be fooled by the word "generalized," because I guarantee you that at least a couple of the nuggets below will be new to you. Let's dive in.

Forget What You Learned as a Kid

Let's start with what you learned as a child. I'm in my midforties, which means growing up in the eighties I watched my parents switch our groceries to every version of fat-free there was. Out was butter, and in came I Can't Believe It's Not Butter. No more heavy cream in the coffee, instead it was Coffee Mate. Bye-bye eggs, time to switch to Egg Beaters. Our homes were suddenly inundated with processed, low/no fat, low/no taste foodlike substances instead of the kitchen staples we had been using for generations.

And what happened to our waistlines? Nothing good, that's for sure. As Big Agra started moving toward selling us processed oils, trans fats, sugared-up everything, and grains galore, Americans saw their dress and pant sizes go up exponentially. Below is a graph of the average American's BMI (body mass index) since 1975. Right before I was born, only about 12 percent of us were obese. By the time I was graduating college, that number had doubled! This chart stopped in 2016, but by then, well over one-third of Americans were not just overweight but obese. That is a sad state of affairs. ***Clearly, we started doing something really, really wrong!***

Clearly, we started doing something really, really wrong!

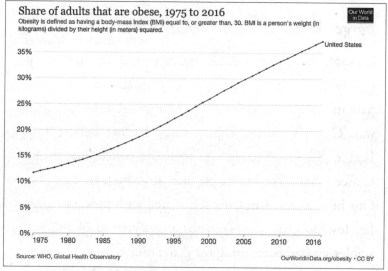

Share of adults that are obese, 1975 to 2016

Obesity is defined as having a body-mass index (BMI) equal to, or greater than, 30. BMI is a person's weight (in kilograms) divided by their height (in meters) squared.

Source: WHO, Global Health Observatory — OurWorldInData.org/obesity · CC BY

Max Roser, Our World in Data, https://ourworldindata.org /grapher/share-of-adults-defined-as-obese, CC BY-SA 3.0, https://commons.wikimedia.org/w/index.php?curid=115295343

Just as we were watching our friends and family gain more and more weight, we were still being taught in school and at home that we should be avoiding fat and eating more grains. There are so many problems with this new way of thinking about nutrition that it is kind of hard to even know where to begin. To avoid going down a history lesson rabbit hole, I'm going to stick with the basic premise that is missing here: why?

Why would it be that in 1977, the US government's Dietary Guidelines for Americans suddenly switched to encouraging us to eat low-fat?[1] Until this point, the USDA recommendations were based on nutrient density. During World War II, recommendations were broken up into seven basic categories to make sure people ate and ate well.

However, in 1956 and through 1992, this was simplified into just four food groups: milk, meat, fruits and vegetables, and bread and cereals.[2] Since we weren't in wartime food scarcity anymore, the government assumed Americans would eat more than enough. This guide was designed to make sure we met our basic nutritional needs.[3] Unfortunately, as the science continued to get muddled on the causes of obesity and heart disease, the USDA decided it needed to be much more specific on exactly what we should be eating. Please read *The Big Fat Surprise* by Nina Teicholz for a detailed history of how this all came to be. But know that, based on the quite flawed idea that all fat is bad, the new dietary guidelines urged us to eat those "healthy whole grains" to the tune of about

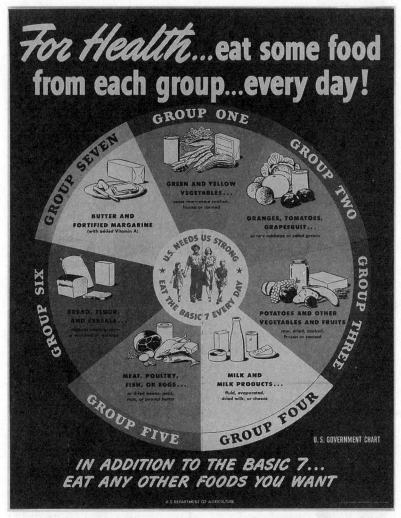

"History of USDA Nutrition Guidelines," Wikipedia, September 9, 2022,
https://en.wikipedia.org/wiki/History_of_USDA_nutrition_guidelines.

six to eleven servings per day and to minimize fat intake at
all costs.[4] Notice the quite stark difference in the food guide
pyramid on the next page in contrast to the "Basic 7" above.

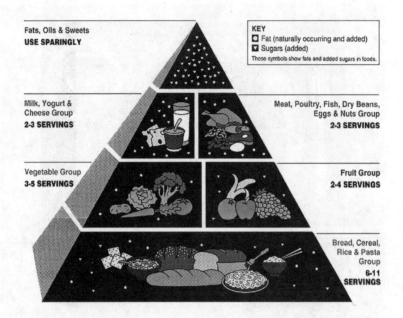

By the food pyramid, from http://www.nal.usda.gov/fnic/Fpyr/pyramid.gif, Public Domain, https://commons.wikimedia.org/w/index.php?curid=680809

Finally, in 2011, this evolved to "My Plate." The idea was shepherded by First Lady Michelle Obama and Tom Vilsack, secretary of agriculture.[5] Although this format was much easier to follow, you might notice that there are exactly zero references to fat on it. And yes, there might be some fat in your protein and dairy choices, but clearly, they didn't want Americans to focus on eating fat at all.

So again, *why?* Let's start with the fact that the US Department of Agriculture was in charge of all this. Their job was to try to keep farmers making money and to sell lots of grains. If this was my goal, I would recommend

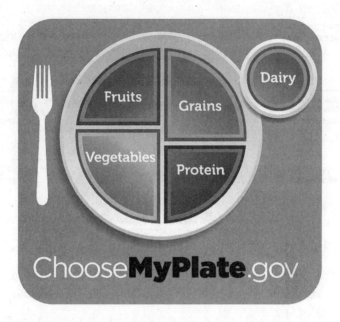

"MyPlate," Wikipedia, July 25, 2022, https://en.wikipedia.org/wiki/MyPlate

everyone eat this way too. The major problem is that it is not in the best interest of the American people's health!

As an adult, I certainly don't pay much attention to what the government may think I should be eating for breakfast, lunch, and dinner, but they still teach it in school. My daughter comes home occasionally with information sheets about diet and nutrition. In school, they tell her to be active and play outside every day, but they also tell her to drink her orange juice, get some "healthy" cereal for breakfast, a nutritious sandwich for lunch, and finish it all off with a bowl of pasta at night. Of course, they recommend she drink her milk, get her fruits and veggies in, and eat her protein, but that is about the extent of the helpful advice they are passing on to my little one's very impressionable mind.

So, let's spend some time doing some critical thinking here on how we can base our own food choices on what is best for our health. None of us have a grain deficiency! I've never heard a doctor say, "You know what you need? More pasta." Uh, no. Many of us, however, have vitamin and mineral deficiencies, protein deficiencies, and even deficiencies in healthy fats. Regardless of your specific goals, few of us have room in our diets for empty calories: for foods that are not chock-full of nutrients. *Every bit of food you take in should add to your overall health, not take away from it.*

> Every bit of food you take in should add to your overall health, not take away from it.

I once heard Dr. Nasha Winters speak at a conference. She is a brilliant expert in natural medicine and mostly speaks to other practitioners about integrative cancer care and research. Dr. Winters (or Dr. Nasha as she prefers) came up with her own "perfect plate" that is leaps and bounds better than anything the USDA has ever put out. In the following picture, you'll see that at least half the plate is filled with produce. Protein is portioned like an accompaniment, fats figure prominently enough to add flavor and satiety, and sweets are an afterthought. If this plate was indicative of what we were teaching our children to eat, the adult population in the US would be infinitely healthier than we are.

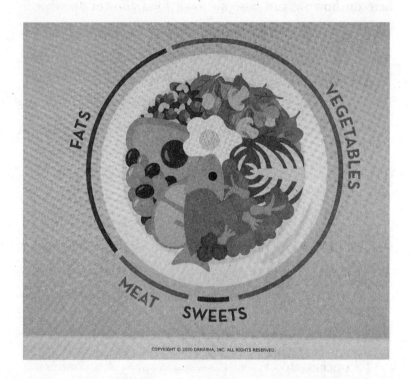

Obesity Is a Disease of Undernourishment

People get in trouble thinking that our physiology has caught up to our technology. Over the last hundred years, food scarcity has become a thing of the past in most developed nations. Anyone who has the means to be reading this book is likely not scavenging for their next meal or worried about how to ration portions through the winter! We refrigerate our food, have chemicals to preserve it way beyond nature's intended shelf life, and can pretty much get anything we crave delivered to our doorstep within minutes. While food scarcity still exists in many areas and cultures, our culinary menu is nothing like that of our great-grandparents. And yet, just like we don't differ much in appearance from their generation, neither does our metabolism.

Our bodies are designed to function under the assumption that food might be scarce. Humans evolved in a time when food needed to be eaten quickly when procured and even gorged on. Our genes know to store the extra calories from a feast in the form of fat on our hips and bellies for use at a later date when starvation sets in. Feast and famine are innate to the human experience. And yet nowadays, we live more in a feast or feast state every day.

There's a good reason why we want to reach for the super sweet goodness of cookies or cake. Nature has taught us over the millennia that all sweet yumminess means there is a lot of nutrition packed in there! Having the treat of a honeycomb or tripping on some berries not yet foraged by animals would have been a windfall in our days as hunters and gatherers. And while today's sugar-laden treats resemble very little nutritionally to that of natural honey or berries, our taste buds don't know the difference. Where we run into trouble is thinking that because it tastes sweet, we should have more.

However, regardless of what our smell and taste tell us, once we ingest that piece of candy or cookie, the lack of vitamins, minerals, and fiber is quickly discovered downstream. Often the sugar is broken down by enzymes right in our mouths, and so quickly that the sugar jolts into our bloodstream without even needing to hit the stomach. What does end up needing to be digested further is done so at such a speed that the body never registers satiety. With little to no fiber, those processed sugars are quickly dispersed into our system and then burned as energy or stored as fat. With that quick burn rate, there's no wonder you are left hungry for more!

This is what I mean when I say obesity is a disease of undernourishment. Remember, we should think of food and nutrition as nourishment. What are you providing your body that will help it to thrive? How is what you are taking into your body supporting your goals? With each taste of something scrumptious, you are making a promise to your body of nutrients coming in. But when it's all digested and processed, and no nutrients come, it makes you infinitely hungry for more! More, more, more! But not more of the same; more of what you had already promised

Eating processed, nutrient-defunct food is basically like lying to yourself!

to feed yourself. *Eating processed, nutrient-defunct foods is basically like lying to yourself!*

When I see people who are not just overweight but obese, I know instantly that there is a disconnect between what is perceived as a good food choice and what their bodies actually need. This problem is greatly compounded by those who do not have the means to buy high-quality food but are instead at the mercy of just buying whatever they can afford. One of the saddest things about the development of the food industry over the last century has been the decline in the quality and quantity of nutrients in the cheapest foods. It seems criminal to me that it's cheaper to get my daughter a soda, fries, and chicken nuggets than it is to get her a glass of milk, corn on the cob, green beans, and a chicken leg. And if I were in a situation where I could have the milkshake, fries, and nuggets for only $3 versus $12, you bet I would make the same choice so many are forced to.

Not only do we struggle to make food choices based on nourishment but we are also teaching a whole generation of children that quick, fast, and tasty is the way to go. Obesity is prevalent not only in adults nowadays but in children! In my 1983 kindergarten class, there was exactly one overweight child. I still remember her name. Not because I am a jerk but because it was so unusual back then that she was an outlier. And when I look back at that class picture, she wasn't even heavy compared to today's standards. Between our lack of activity with so much technology at our fingertips and our overabundance of quickly attained, calorie-laden, under-nourishing foods, it's a wonder that every child isn't dealing with obesity.

Don't Teach Your Kids What You Were Taught

Even doing what I do for a living, I struggle with providing my daughter with the tools she needs to be healthy. At the time of this writing, we are rounding out the second year of the COVID-19 pandemic. When school got shut down, she was in the spring semester of third grade. Suddenly she and most every other child went from being nonstop moving whirlwinds all day to being stuck at home in front of a screen. No PE, no organized sports, no playdates. Instead of sched-uled mealtimes, she was home all day with access to the kitchen whenever she craved a treat.

Regardless of having a health coach for a mom, my little one suddenly found herself putting on weight beyond what she'd ever experienced. It took me almost a year to realize what was happening right before my eyes! She started to be aware of the changes herself and wasn't happy about it. We had to have a conversation about structured mealtimes, eating at the table with no screens, and getting outdoor activity every day. Luckily she is self-aware enough to know it was time and the right thing to do. Within six months, she had not gained any weight despite growing about two inches, was back in school with her friends, and felt like the vibrant, happy child she should be.

What a lesson that was for me! And I won't lie; it was really hard for me to have that chat with her about choosing healthy foods, not eating distractedly, and getting movement every day. It was hard because when I was just a little older than she was, I started paying way too much attention to how I looked, and how thin I was, and I started comparing myself to others. Since the day she was born, I have sworn I would do everything in my power to prevent her from dealing with disordered eating as I did in my adolescence. And yet here I was, having to tell my daughter that she needed to watch what she was eating! Agony, I tell you. Luckily, it was all set in the context of every other person (seemingly in the whole world) dealing with the same issue: the COVID-19-LBS!

But even without a pandemic, teaching and modeling healthy eating for our children is not easy. When most of us have spent a good portion of our adult lives dealing with food-related issues of some sort, how can we possibly model a healthy relationship with food for our progeny? Let's start by looking at the things we know didn't work for us growing up:

- Being stuck at the table until your plate was clean
- Being told not to waste food because starving children somewhere would love to have it
- Watching our parents follow the latest diet craze
- Comparing ourselves to impossible standards of beauty in the media

"Finish your food, or you won't be leaving this table!" Oh boy, I remember my little brother being stuck at that table for what seemed like hours when he wouldn't finish his vegetables. I'm sure it was more like thirty minutes, but to little kids, it was an eternity. I also remember that we had this little space under the table where the table leaves fit in and where my brother and I would hide food when we just couldn't stomach another bite. Oh, the look of horror when my mother would go to put a table leaf in and find the moldy peas and zucchini left there from who knows how many months ago!

You'll notice I didn't say that I was the one left at the table—nope. I'm not sure if that was because I'm a girl, and therefore wiping my plate clean was not expected, or because I was such a "good girl" that I just ate it all to avoid punishment. I was always a pleaser and relished the fact that my brother was always the one getting in trouble! I'll go into more about this later, but for now, just know that being a perfectionist and pleaser was not going to help me in the ensuing years (health-wise).

"Don't you know there are starving children in this world? You need to clean that plate!" There's no doubt that food insecurity runs rampant throughout the world, but there's no fixing that by making your kid clean their plate.

Let's be serious, does your wallet know if that food got eaten or not?

I think we were told that instead of what our parents (or now we as adults) were really thinking: "I don't want to waste any more money on food you don't eat!" *Let's be serious, does your wallet know if that food got eaten or not?* Your bank account doesn't care whether the leftovers ended up in your kids' bellies, the trash, a storage bag, or your rear end. If we're going to be successful in managing our own food intake and modeling good behaviors for our children, we have to let go of the "clean plate" idea once and for all!

If your kids are consistently leaving food on their plates, then serve them smaller portions. They can always get more when they finish. If you find yourself cleaning their plates with your mouth, STOP! This is the number one way I get parents to drop a quick five to ten pounds. Those little nibbles of leftover snacks and meals add up to serious extra calories. What's more, you aren't registering satiety or fullness from those nibbles. So, suddenly, you have hundreds of extra calories you are taking in every day—all in the name of not wasting food. It can become a serious barrier to your long-term goals.

The most detrimental thing about the "clean plate" mindset is that it totally disrupts your body's ability to understand true fullness and hunger. Children have these wonderfully, fully functional hormones that signal things like, "You're hungry; you should eat." "You're getting full; slow down." And, "You're full now; time to do something else." But as we get told over and over again to eat meals at dictated times and not stop eating until our plates are clean, this signaling gets dampened. The digestive system, brain, and hormones all keep sending these signals, but when we don't listen to them and we over-ride what they are telling us to do, those signals stop working altogether.

When my daughter was about four years old, we would occasionally go to this local creamery for the most delectable ice cream. She would beg me to take her, then hem and haw over which combination of flavors to pick for her scoops. After

> The most detrimental thing about the "clean plate" mindest is that it totally disrupts your body's ability to understand true fullness and hunger.

we sat down and started digging in with "oohs" and "yums," she would quickly start getting distracted and begin running around. Then I'd ask if she was done, and she'd look at me as if to say, "With what?" She was totally over the ice cream at that point and ready to move on. Have you ever seen an adult sit down to a much-anticipated dessert and then walk away after three bites? I never have! It's infuriating when you just shelled out six dollars for some gourmet small-batch ice cream, but such is life. My wallet has already been hit. Why should I add insult to injury by adding those uneaten calories to my hips?

"I'm going keto." Or vegan, or Zone, or Mediterranean, or whatever. I watched my father jump head-first into the low-fat craze in the late eighties and early nineties. Instead of having one delicious chocolate chip cookie, he'd have a whole sleeve of fat-free Joseph's or Snackwell's. Our Klondike bars were replaced with low-fat ice cream. This certainly didn't make weight loss easier for him, nor did it mean he could go to fewer aerobics classes. It didn't help him, and it certainly didn't help me either.

I was always watching those around me and trying to extrapolate what works, what doesn't, what's right, what's wrong … I learned that food needs to be controlled, that it shouldn't really taste that good, and that eating delicious things was bad. I didn't want to be fat, and from what I gathered, eating rich foods was going to make me fat! Keep in mind, I'm not blaming my father or anyone for my burgeoning eating disorder, but my point is we have to model for our children and families what it means to nourish oneself, not how to diet down!

You Should Love Everything You Eat!

No, really. Contrary to what I surmised as a kid, what is the purpose of trying to adhere to a diet or plan that isn't enjoyable? Unless you are stuck in a situation where food is hard to come by, there is *no* reason to settle for anything less than delicious. In fact, humans have an innate attraction to yummy foods because that usually means they are also loaded with nutrients essential to our health. When we would procure fresh honey, berries in a field, or ripe stone fruit, you can bet we'd gorge ourselves on that natural sugar. But it wasn't the sugar alone our ancestors wanted, it was all the vitamins and minerals in those foods that would help them fight off disease and add to their vitality. Like I said before, just because our technology has found ways to make processed foods that are loaded with that sweet taste but none of the upsides of nutrition, it doesn't mean our taste buds know the difference.

Not only should the food you choose to put in your mouth be delicious, but it should also be nutritious (nourishing). When we decided to eschew foods like butter, eggs, and cream, we ended up trading them in for fat-free foodlike versions that were devoid of both nutrients and taste! What were we thinking? When my family started stocking fat-free milk in the fridge as a kid, I thought that I just didn't like milk.

I never drank the stuff unless it was to drench my cereal. It tasted like white water to me and was just not good. Decades later, as an adult, I finally tried cream top milk. Oh-my-Lord! I don't know if you have ever tasted that goodness, but holy moly, it's kind of magical! I might have drunk gallons of the stuff as a kid if that had been on the menu.

When you get the chance to taste real food, it is truly the best! Real, unadulterated, back to basics, like nature intended, is the nourishment our bodies both need and crave. It can be kind of a shock to the system at first. I've had many clients who are so indoctrinated into the low-fat, low-cholesterol, low-salt, low-flavor dogma we've been "fed" all these years that they almost can't even believe I'm telling them to go and add fat to their diet! Like, "Wait, eggs are not going to kill me?" "Butter is not the devil incarnate?" "Beef won't make me fat?" Seriously, we have lost all sight of what food is and what it is for.

> You are taking something from your enviroment and PUTTING IT IN YOUR BODY.

For just a second, I want you to think about what "eating" really is. *You are taking something from your environment and PUTTING IT IN YOUR BODY.* Let me say that again, PUTTING IT IN YOUR BODY!

Is there literally anything else in this world that you put *in* your body and do not think a little bit about first? And yet so many people seem to be surprised when they realize that what they have been taking in is causing health issues. Food is not innocuous. It can be very powerful in its effects.

Food is nourishment:

- Proteins: for building muscle, assisting in every metabolic function at the cellular level, and feeding chemicals for brain function.

- Fats: for keeping hormones functioning optimally, for a dense source of energy, for organ function, and for help in absorbing minerals and fat-soluble vitamins.

- Fiber: for proper digestion, for seeding healthy microorganisms in our gut.

- Minerals: for proper cellular function and metabolism, for strong bones, for healthy skin, hair, and so on.

- Vitamins: for a healthy immune system and general function of every cell in the body.

With overprocessed foodlike substances, we don't get much of these things. You might get a few man-made vitamins thrown back in, but they won't be in the most usable form. Not only did Mother Nature put all the goodies we need into natural food but she also put them into the perfect combinations for us to be able to completely nourish ourselves. Did you know that you can't absorb calcium, magnesium, phosphorus, vitamin D, or any other goodie you should get from a glass of milk if there's not enough fat in it? Yep. All of those are fat-soluble minerals and vitamins. That means no fat, and no vitamins for you. Nada.

Aside from being defunct in nutrients, processed foods are addictive. Food producers have figured out how to use our own physiology against us. They have food scientists that work to make sure they find a "bliss point" where the flavors light up your brain, just like it would react to drugs! I learned this term by reading *Salt Sugar Fat: How the Food Giants Hooked Us* by Michael Moss. He does a deep dive into how food scientists use brain chemistry, hormones, and science to get us hooked on their products. Not only do we end up overeating these foods; they are also still deficient in the nutrients our bodies need to thrive. That is why we end up going back to the cupboard for more and more and more! When I told you earlier that obesity is a disease of undernourishment, this is exactly what I was talking about.

When I say that you need to love what you eat, I don't mean that you get to eat Doritos and pizza whenever you want. I mean that you get to eat whole foods, with all the natural fats and flavors that nature intended, and savor every bite. When you sit down to a meal, it should look, smell, and taste delicious. I will help you figure out how to find what foods work for you and what foods don't. I will help you make choices on what to eat and what to avoid based on your preferences and your goals.

It's my goal to help you find a way to nourish yourself today and throughout your life.

If you don't enjoy your meals, you won't stick with them. *It's my goal to help you find a way to nourish yourself today and throughout your life.* Although food fads will come and go, and diet trends and food technology will evolve, if you always come back to these principles, you will be successful in both attaining and sustaining your goals. There is no point in signing up to make changes to your diet if it is not something you can do over the long term. Why bother doing a juice fast that will leave you starved and depleted and likely devouring every morsel in the cupboard the day it is done? Why make yourself eat meal replacements, powders, and other strange-colored tinctures if you can't possibly figure out how to eat when you are with friends and family? You can eat healthfully, nourish yourself, attain your goals, *and* enjoy the ride!

Love what you eat, but food is not your lover. You should enjoy your food for all it is: nourishing, sustaining, and life-giving. But:

Food is not your friend.
Food is not your lover.
Food is not a pastime.
Food is not a therapist.
Food is not entertainment.
Food is not your crutch.

Coming to terms not only with what you are choosing to eat but *why* is essential to your long-term success!

Don't Eat If You're Not Hungry. Period.

This is one of the hardest things to teach people. When I advise my clients not to eat until they are truly hungry, it sounds like sacrilege. We have had it ingrained in us since a very young age that we need to "eat a good breakfast." We have been taught that all celebrations revolve around food. Food is love. Food is a reward. "Have a snack." "Don't offend your host; you must eat whatever is served." "Don't you want seconds?" And of course, "Don't leave food on that plate; it needs to be cleaned before you leave the table."

While I certainly wouldn't want you to offend Grandma by not having a slice of her famous pie, those indulgences are both worth it and should be exceptions, not the norm. Tapping into your hunger and satiety cues is not as easy as you'd think. Remember earlier when I told you about how frustrating it is to see a kid waste the better part of an overpriced ice cream cone? That is a young body and hormone system that still knows true hunger and true fullness.

When we are constantly eating on a schedule, cleaning our plates out of habit, snacking mindlessly, and using food as a reward, we eventually lose the ability to hear the signals our body is sending. Our ancestors didn't have to log their food into an app to see how many calories they had left to eat in a day. But they also didn't have refrigeration and preservatives that allowed them to have snacks any time they wanted. *Almost every adult I have ever worked with has lost track of what was once an innate human function: knowing when they are hungry.*

Almost every adult I have ever worked with has lost track of what was once an innate human function: knowing when they are hungry.

Our hunger and fullness signals, when working properly, are quite elegant and precise. Starting with the first bite of food you take, peristalsis (the wavelike movements of muscles through your digestive tract) starts. This signals the stomach to get the digestive juices flowing. Once the stomach is full enough, that change in volume signals to your brain that it's time to stop shoveling food into your piehole. Once all the food has been digested and moved into the colon, if you don't have a ton of extra body fat around, you'll sense a signal that it's time to start looking for food again. If you do have some extra pounds on you, your body would start mobilizing all those extra calories to burn for energy.

Unfortunately, many people don't know what true hunger feels like anymore. Nor do they eat slowly and with enough presence to sense when they should put the fork down. And almost everyone has enough stored calories on their bums or bellies to be able to go days without food if only they'd allow themselves the chance to start burning them off.

When you give yourself the breadth to just wait—to not eat—that is when you start to turn the signaling back on. It's not easy. And trust me, during this pandemic, work-from-home, ooh the kitchen is just next-door state we've all been in, it has even been a struggle for me to keep my meals from turning into twenty-four snacks. Those days when I give into temptation: a little nibble between breakfast and lunch, and then a little pre-lunch, and then something yummy after lunch … It's a disaster. I end up with my head all scrambled. I have no idea what I have eaten. I am never hungry and never full. I go to bed feeling annoyed with myself. And I do this for a living!

The only antidote to the snack all-day habit we seem to get ourselves into is to stop. Just stop. Try it out on a weekend day when you don't have any meal-related commitments. Here's your plan:

- When you wake up, drink a full glass of water first thing (well after you tinkle). But before coffee or anything else.

- Then start doing something, anything. Read the news, take a walk, make love, work out, meditate, whatever. Just get going on something.

- Just listen. Listen to your body's signals of hunger. When you first notice it, is it because this is the time you always eat? Or are you really hungry? If you don't know, wait a few more minutes.

- When you decide to eat, do it with intention. Plan out what you will put on your plate. Make it look nice. Sit down away from the kitchen counter and with all devices off (unless they are playing music).

- As you eat, notice: How does your food taste? Do you like the combination of foods you picked? Are you getting full? If you're not full, do you need more? More of what?

- When you start to feel full, is it really fullness, or is it boredom? Put your fork down and wait a minute before you decide.

- Put the plate away and leave the kitchen.

- Repeat this process for every meal that day.

At the end of your weekend experiment (or even during), take some notes on how you feel at each point. Below is a little worksheet for you to kind of map out your experience. As you become more comfortable with the process, you will find that it is quite liberating. You don't end up thinking about food all day long. You aren't consumed by it (pun intended). The fear of being hungry just goes away. I mean, really, what is the worst that can happen if you get hungry? You're not a child. You're not going to pass out or crash the car. You're just hungry. The worst that could happen is you might tap into your fat stores for energy and finally start burning off that gut!

Eat When You're Hungry Experiment Notes

Event	Hunger Before	Fullness After	Notes
Wake up, drink water			
Do something first			
Breakfast			
Between breakfast and lunch			
Lunch			
Between lunch and dinner			
Dinner			
After dinner			

"Mindful Eating": An Overused but Critical Term

The weekend experiment of eating only when you're hungry works only if you are really paying attention to your body's signals and being present and appreciative of what you're eating. I hear the term "mindful eating" thrown around the blogosphere quite often. I understand the term, as do most, but it also sort of dismisses the practice as something airy-fairy and done only by those who meditate daily and do tai chi in the morning. Not at all. Being present and aware of your intake is critical to your success in getting and keeping excess weight off. I would go so far as to say that if you did *nothing* else to change your eating habits, this one thing could make a difference in your long-term health more than any other change. I mean it! More than exercise, more than eating your veggies. ***Being fully engaged and focused on your food is the number one thing that could keep you from ever worrying about your weight again.***

Being fully engaged and focused on your food is the number one thing that could keep you from ever worrying about your weight again.

Okay, so that is a bold claim, I know. But think for a minute about all the various times you've found yourself overconsuming. What are the settings? Were you hovering over the kitchen counter? Did you scoop food right out of the container while no one was looking? Were you watching TV? At your desk parsing through emails? Scrolling on social media? In your car from point A to B? Lying in bed bingeing the latest series? For me, the answers are yes, yes, yes, yes, yes, yes, and yes. What was your state of mind when you overate in the past? Distracted? Lonely? Stressed? Anxious? Tired? Overwhelmed? Yes, yes, yes, yes, yes, and yes.

Every one of those times you nibbled your way through a TV series, mindlessly polished off a bag of chips while scrolling social media, or scooped ice cream into your mouth while fretting about relationship stress, you were adding extra (and empty) calories to your waistline. And don't think that these noshes are just little snacks that won't impact you over time. I'm pretty sure you can polish off thousands of calories when you're unaware. Don't believe me? Do you know that a regular bag of popcorn (not a large or jumbo, mind you) tops out at 600 calories? And that's before you add butter. How many of us can even get full after that? Not many. It's usually followed by dinner or comes after dinner, and maybe a few bites of your friend's candy. You do that once a week and you've already gained a pound that month! Can you imagine if you had to eat the same bag of popcorn while sitting at the table with nothing to watch? Would you even finish half of it?

That's not to say you should never have popcorn at the movies again, but you have to factor it into your day. If you know you are going to a movie and like to have popcorn, maybe you have a small dinner before and choose the child's size popcorn instead. Being aware requires you to also plan. Think about what you had for breakfast, for lunch. Have you had snacks today? Are you really hungry? Once you've done the weekend experiment a few times, start trying it during the week. Slowly start bringing that practice into your everyday.

When you become more comfortable with only eating when you are hungry, you can get more detailed with your mindfulness around your eating. Here are my favorite ways to make sure each and every bite of food I eat is not only enjoyed but that my body gets the signal that it has nourishment, is ready to start digesting, and won't be hungry again for hours:

- No standing up.
- Aggregate your food onto one plate.
- No snacks.
- No screens.
- No other activity.
- Take three breaths first.
- Have all the components: protein, fat, and produce.
- Make it pretty, and even fun.
- Leave the eating area, kitchen, or pantry when done.

- Keep alcohol separate.
- Pick your poison.
- Eat with your nondominant hand.

No standing up. This is a big one. Unless you are at a cocktail party or somewhere that doesn't offer chairs, do not eat standing up. The simple act of sitting down with a plate in front of you signals that you are about to start eating. If you are standing up while noshing, chances are you are nibbling (not having a real meal) and therefore won't register any satisfaction from whatever you're putting in your mouth. This also directly cuts back on the snacks you'll consume while making dinner, putting together premade lunches, or whatever. You know that nibbling you do when no one is looking—the kind when you scoop peanut butter or ice cream straight out of the container? It's really hard to overeat when you force yourself to take a seat!

Aggregate your food onto one plate. This is a great tip to use when you're at an event. Anytime there's a buffet table or hors d'oeuvres being passed around, this is my number one go-to move. Grab a plate and purposefully start choosing your foods. Make sure to get at least one of each thing you just don't want to pass up. If you have to wait for servers to come around with something special, wait. If you're at a buffet, put all the things you want onto that plate and know that there's *no* going back! You get only one pass at it. Do your absolute best to get all you need onto that one plate. If you must go back for seconds, do so only after you have given yourself ten minutes or more to make sure you're still hungry, and know what you are going to grab before you go.

By looking at your food, all mounded into one heap on a plate, you have a much better idea of all that you've consumed. If, instead, you have an hors d'oeuvre here, another there, a few bites from this, a few more from that, you have no idea how much you have eaten. This also takes you back to being aware of how full and hungry you are. Having a meal—all your food on one plate—allows you to assess how hungry or full you are once you've finished eating. There needs to be a start and stop to the eating, not a constant flow. This applies at home too. If you took each nibble you had from your kids' plates, while cooking, while unpacking groceries, and put them all together before you stuck them in your mouth, you'd be astonished—and likely quite embarrassed. So don't do it.

No snacks. If you are planning your meals out with intent and with keeping your long-term goals in mind, snacking should not be in the mix. I will dig deeper into how to plan out your meals based on your goals below, but for now, know that if you make sure to aggregate your food onto one plate, and are fully present, you should get full enough to go three to four hours (or more) before the next meal. If you can't, then something was missing from the previous meal. Meals should be satisfying and give you the breadth to not even think about food for hours afterward!

I can't tell you how many women (sorry, it's true, this is

Fullness means you have no more cravings and that you have control.

mostly a female issue) I have had to tell to eat more. When I tell them to increase the size of their meals by 25–50 percent, they look at me like I'm nuts! But guess what happens? They stop snacking. Like, immediately! It's an instantaneous fix. If you are one of those people who sort of noshes their way through the day (a grazer), you need to pay attention right here. You are doing yourself no favors by nibbling all day. Start right now—the next time you eat. Put a *meal* together, sit down, and get full. Don't be scared to get full. It's okay. *Fullness means you have no more cravings and that you have control.*

I say this is a predominantly female issue because it seems that so many of us have been taught that it's gross to be full. It's like having our stomach actually reach capacity is a bad thing. Only dudes eat like that. I call bullshit! Every man I know can sit down to a giant meal, get stuffed, and then sometimes not eat for like an entire day. I know very few, if any, women who can do this. We just have a few bites, say we are "good," and then end up scraping the edges of the ice cream bin thirty minutes later. No more! Get full, ladies!

No screens. This is a really hard habit to break. So many of us, especially when eating alone, will pop the news on, start scrolling through social media, or catch up on emails at our desks while eating. Please *stop!* Today. I told my daughter that if she wanted to never worry about her weight, all she has to do is not eat in front of a screen. Period. How many times have you found yourself at the end of something delicious while catching up on Netflix, or watching a movie, and thought, "Wow, I already ate all that?" That's not good. That means that not only did your brain not register all the food you just consumed but neither did your digestive system.

If you take the above rules and add the "no screens" to them, this is the scene: You are starting to get hungry for lunch. Maybe you're in a meeting and sense your tummy rumbling. Instead of reaching for a snack in your desk drawer, you have a few sips of water and hold off until the meeting ends. You get up and go to the cafeteria or kitchen and amass some protein, some veggies, maybe a little potato on the side, and drizzle some olive oil over it all. Then you find a nice place to sit near the window; somewhere you can watch nature or even people strolling by. Maybe you put your earphones in and listen to some music. You look down at the beautiful meal you've laid out and start enjoying. It smells good, tastes good, and each bite is delicious. But then, somewhere about two-thirds of the way through your meal, your stomach is getting full. You're tired of looking out the window, and realizing you have another meeting starting in a few minutes, you push away from the table, grab a to-go box for your leftovers, and get back to the grind.

Wouldn't it be nice to just step away like that? It's okay that you get bored eating a meal and not get distracted by something on a screen. This allows your mind and body to take in your meal, appreciate it, digest it well, and feel satisfied for hours to come.

No other activity. This falls in line with the above advice to not eat in front of a screen. But it goes a bit further. While it's fine, and even more enjoyable to eat with friends or family at the table and engage in conversation, more distracting activities are a problem when it comes to registering hunger and fullness. Eating in your car is a big one. Please don't do this. First of all, it usually entails snacking, which we have already discussed. If you have a lot of travel time in your day, make sure that the meal before and after your travel time is substantial. Secondly, but more importantly, you will (I hope) be so focused on the road that the food won't be noticed or appreciated. Also, car food is usually junk food. So just don't.

There's also eating while working, eating while reading, and eating while doing pretty much anything besides enjoying your company at the table. Anything that moves your eyes and mental focus away from appreciating your meal is a no-go.

Take three breaths first. I'm not a particularly religious person. However, I think the act of saying grace or a prayer before a meal is a wonderful practice. When I sit down for my meal, even if I am with others, I like to just take three slow breaths before I dig in. You don't have to be weird about it and get everyone's attention. Just look at your plate, breathe in slowly, exhale, and repeat twice more. Then pick up your fork or spoon and get rolling. That little pause has a huge impact. It can be a signal to your digestive system: "Hey, you smell that? Look at what's headed your way, belly!"

At first, it can be hard to remember to do this. But once you get in the habit, I think you'll get to enjoy this bit. It is also a good check on yourself: Is the meal I chose what I really want? Is this healthy? How hungry am I? Will this be enough to satisfy me? Inserting a pause is a great way to stay on track regardless of your goals with health, challenges with food, and current situation.

Have all the components: protein, fat, and produce. You can't make a meal out of one or two ingredients. I know you may think you can, but not really. A meal needs to have these three critical components to both satisfy and nourish you. With just one missing piece, you may find yourself having cravings for more, feeling unsatisfied, and reaching for snacks shortly after you eat. *Set yourself up for success by having protein, fat, and produce every time you fix a meal.*

Protein, and the amino acids we

Set yourself up for success by having protein, fat, and produce every time you fix a meal.

get from it, are critical to feeling and staying full. They burn slowly and keep blood sugar stable. Protein, be it animal protein, or even plant protein, helps keep our muscles strong, gives us the building blocks for neurotransmitters for clear thinking and a stable mood, and is necessary for all the cells in our body to function optimally. While sources of protein from animals will give you the most complete amino acid profile, you can get really close if using supplemental plant protein like pea and hemp. Soy, in particular soy protein isolate, can be an issue in regard to hormone and thyroid health. This topic is beyond the scope of this book, but for further reading, check out *The Whole Soy Story* by Kaayla T. Daniel.

Fat, contrary to what many might believe, is quite necessary for our diets. I am personally not afraid of saturated fats, and to be honest, the current science does not support the idea that they will kill you. The only fats I would caution you to avoid are processed fats like canola oil, sunflower oil, safflower oil, and so on. You can read more on this topic at Dr. Cate Shanahan's website: www. DrCate.com. For now, just know that without enough fat in your meal, you won't be able to properly absorb fat-soluble vitamins and minerals. Things like phosphorus, calcium, magnesium, vitamin A, vitamin D, and many more all need a little fat to be properly absorbed and assimilated into your system. Fats in your meal will also help keep you satisfied longer because they digest more slowly. Healthy fats like avocado, olives, and fish will help with a healthy gut, great skin, and overall nourishment.

Produce should be a no-brainer, but so many of us do not get enough in our day. This is where the magic happens. By making sure you get varied vegetables and fruits, you will add to your diet all the complements of vitamins and minerals, fiber and starch, and so much flavor. The easiest way to do this is to make sure each meal has some vibrant color. Maybe breakfast has seasonal berries in bright blue or red, then lunch has some deep green colored leafies and some bright yellow from bell pepper or heirloom tomatoes. Dinner might even have more colors: orange from potato or carrot, white from fennel or onion, and varied hues of green. If you just focus on getting colors of all types into your meals, you won't have to spend time figuring out what is missing from your diet—you'll have gotten a broad spectrum of vitamins, minerals, and fiber that is beyond your ability to count.

When it comes to mindfulness, you'll be surprised that having a pretty plate with a lot of colors helps you enjoy your meal more. The added fiber and volume from produce will help you feel full sooner and for longer.

Make it pretty and even fun. Rolling straight from our colorful plate idea, don't forget to make your food enjoyable to consume. If you're going to take the time to put all the components of your meal onto one plate, which you should, you might as well take a few seconds to make it pretty. That might just mean using some of your good plates instead of an old one. It might mean that you sit down with a candle or some nice music in the background. Maybe you have others you're eating with, and you take a minute to make sure the table is set nicely. If you have younger ones around the house, it's fun to make silly faces or scenes with your food. What matters is that you sit down to a meal that you truly enjoy!

Leave the eating area when you're done. Boy, this is so important! I could almost write a whole chapter about how critical this is to succeed in being mindful of what you eat. Once you decide that you're done eating, put the plate away. Then, without hesitation, leave the eating area. Even if you have to come back later to clean up the kitchen or something, give yourself about twenty minutes just to let it sit with you first. It will take that long for your hormones and digestion to signal how full you are. If, after that, you still really need something to top you off, do so with a plan. Grab what you need, put it on another plate, and force yourself to sit down. Do not have that after-dinner snack standing in the kitchen or pantry. The same rule applies to parties and other people's homes. Once you're done eating at a cocktail party, for example, put the plate down and walk further away from where the food is being served to enjoy other company. If at a sit-down dinner, once you've had your fill, turn your utensils down on your plate (a polite signal of being done), and push your plate a few inches from you as you wait for others to finish their meals. The most important thing is that you send your brain and body the clear signal of being done and give yourself the time to physically and mentally get in rest and digest mode.

Keep alcohol separate. This one is a bit controversial, and please know that I'm fully aware you're going to think I'm nuts here, but: drink before you eat. WHAT? Yep, I said that. Now here's why: If you enjoy a cocktail here and there, a glass of wine, and so on, you want it to be enjoyable, maybe take the edge off, but not thwart your fitness efforts. So, don't let it affect your waistline. You want to have those empty calories when your liver glycogen (the liver's form of storing sugar/energy) is at its lowest, and before you top it off with food. If you are already into your meal with that first glass, there is nowhere for those extra calories to go besides straight to your fat stores.

Why does common sense tell us to drink on a full stomach? Well, because you have a lot already in your digestive system, and the alcohol doesn't hit you nearly as fast. While this does make sense from a safety perspective, it actually proves my point. The alcohol doesn't really hit your system, so you might end up drinking even more. If you are a seasoned drinker, you will likely not even feel the effects of one glass of wine during a meal. So you might need two, or three, or even more to get the feel-good vibes you were hoping for. But, assuming you do not need to drive or do other dangerous activities if you have just one glass as you are ordering your food and finish it as your food arrives, you'll find you have a gentle effect that likely will dilute by the end of dinner.

If you are a total lightweight and get tipsy from just the smell of booze, you might want to put this one in your back pocket. Please, use your judgment on when and how to drink. But if you are a regular drinker and know that all those extra calories are starting to negate your fitness goals, this is a great tip. Imagine being able to enjoy just one glass, and that's it. How liberating! And think about all the extra calories you won't be consuming. The average glass of wine has about 140 calories (not a generous pour, BTW), and most straight cocktails are about the same (way higher if a mixed drink). If you go from having a few of those at about 300–600 empty calories a sitting to a mere 140–150, that is a huge dent in your overall intake. The real magic happens when we combine this advice with the next section:

Pick your poisons. I am by no means one of those people who thinks carbs are the devil. However, depending on your goals, empty calories and sugar are just not in most people's best interests. Even those who need to gain weight should avoid too much in the way of sugary drinks, processed carbohydrates, and gooey desserts. For the majority who would like to lose some weight, it is really important to minimize empty calories. You need to pick your poisons!

For example, let's say you are meeting some friends for

a birthday dinner. The restaurant is famous for the birthday dessert tray they bring out for the table. Everything there is going to be scrumptious. So, you know in advance that you're going to have some treats, but you don't want to go nuts. This is where you need to strategize. If you really want to take part in the dessert, then you should probably lay off the booze that night. I'd also suggest you pass on the bread and lay off the extra starch on your plate (rice, pasta, etc.). If you couldn't care less about dessert and would prefer to have a cocktail with your friends, then make a pact not to have the sweets after your inhibitions and judgment are affected by drinking. Do you see my point?

This doesn't apply just to special events, it applies to all kinds of scenarios. Maybe you love going to the baseball game and just have to have a bag of peanuts. Then fine, but make sure to have some veggies earlier in the day (or after), and drink a lot of water instead of beer at the game. Going to the movies and just can't pass on some popcorn? No problem. Just order a small and pass on the candy and soda.

While we are on the topic, let me touch on the question I get year after year over and over and over again: "How can I get through the holidays without gaining weight?" To be brief, the same way you do all the other days. If you just keep the principles that I have laid out for you in this section in mind, you will always be successful. If you don't eat standing up, sit down and aggregate your food into one meal, and step away from the eating area, you're already way ahead of the previous year's mistakes. On top of that, if you think about picking your poisons, you will be less likely to dip into the egg nog, have a heaping pile of stuffing, and have three types of dessert after. It's not like all these guidelines go out the window as soon as the holidays arrive. Do yourself the favor of not having to start all over in January (again).

Eat with your nondominant hand. This is a kind of fun yet silly tip, but I swear it can be effective. If you are the kind of person who is done with their meal first every time or inhales your meal so quickly you barely remember what you ate, this is perfect for you.

My father is left-handed, and for some reason, I just always thought that was so cool. As a kid, I was so intrigued by the way he held a pen and how he wrote. Silly, I know. I taught myself to write with my left hand. I would use my obsession with crossword puzzles to practice writing my block letters. Until I got pretty good, I had to slow down and pay attention to each stroke I wrote. Crossing my *T*'s and making the curl of a *Q* was suddenly a real challenge.

As an adult, I have been playing with this idea when it comes to eating with more mindfulness. I'm good enough now that I even eat left-handed in restaurants. But in the beginning, I was really slow, and it was not easy. A small snack would take me twice the time it used to, all because shoveling with a spoon with your nondominant hand is no joke. Heck, even holding a taco can be hard when you're not used to it. I encourage you to try this in conjunction with all the other tips and tricks above. Notice how you have to think about where to put your fingers, how to angle your hand as you reach for your mouth, and how much longer it takes you to finish your food. But as I mentioned earlier, you might want to start in the comfort of your own home before you take this one on the road. ;)

Putting Mindful Eating into Play

I have laid out lots of ideas on ways to start working toward really eating mindfully. These are simple tips, tricks, rules to live by, and just common sense to follow that will reap huge rewards long term. That said, not all of them will work for you. Some will be impossible, and others will be a total hit. Again, my goal is to help you "own your wellness." So let me help you figure out which of these ideas might be the most helpful along this journey. Below is another chart for you to fill out. Next to each mindful eating approach, I have left you room for notes. Try each one by itself for a few days. Set up some sort of cue to remind you to stick with it. Then make notes on how each worked for you. I even left space at the bottom for you to add your own ideas. After getting through each, decide which are keepers and which you might just put in your back pocket for another day.

Mindfulness Habit	#Days Tried	Cue That Helped	Notes
No standing up while eating at all.			
Aggregate food onto one plate.			
No snacks, period.			
No screens while eating.			
No other activity besides conversation or listening to music.			
Take three breaths first, then the first bite.			
Have all the main components: protein, fat, and produce at each meal.			
Make it pretty, and even fun.			
Leave the eating area, kitchen, or pantry when done.			
Keep alcohol separate.			
Pick your poisons.			
Eat with your nondominant hand.			
Other ideas:			

Does It Support Your Goal?

I am confident that eating with the mindfulness practices we discussed earlier will help you get far toward nourishing yourself appropriately. You'll innately make better decisions around food, decisions that will help you get closer and closer to your long-term wellness goals. Of course, mindfulness is only a piece of the puzzle when it comes to reaching that next level. All of your choices when it comes to nourishing yourself have to be in line with your short and long-term goals to work. You have to go back to identifying your "why." This is where you flip back to the section where you laid out your reasons for wanting to optimize your health. You might also want to look back at the notes you made earlier about your vision of your ideal life. Now, let's take both of those together and figure out a solid goal for you.

I'm going to go through general goals you might have, but before you flip forward to the section you think applies to you the most, take a moment to dial into your goals. It's one thing to have a goal and another to have a very specific goal. Please don't just say, "I want to lose weight." How much? By when? If your goal is to get stronger or more toned, again, be specific: What do you mean by stronger? Do you want to do five pull-ups? Do you want to be able to run five miles? Do you want visible definition in your arms and back? What if you just want to manage or prevent chronic disease? Again, which ones? Is arthritis not allowing you to move freely? Does diabetes or heart disease run in your family? Let's nail down your "why" and the goal related to that before you dig into the "how."

On the following page, I lay out some ideas of what could be the "why" behind your goals. I'd like you to look through these and see which resonates with you. Then, take a moment to write down a specific goal to reach (I've given you an example for each). You'll want to keep these in mind for the remainder of this chapter, but we will revisit this in later sections as well. So please don't gloss over this page—this is where you are setting up the framework for all you do in *owning your wellness*.

Once you've taken the time to noodle on each of the goals I lay out for you here, we can start working on how to reach them. Let's spend time delving into strategies around food to help you get where you're trying to go. I will use the generalized goals in the chart to help structure my advice. However, even if your personal goal doesn't necessarily line up with the topic I'm discussing, you may want to peruse that section anyhow. There is a lot of overlap between various goals and the strategies you can employ to achieve them.

General Goal	Specific Goal	Why?	Personal Notes
Weight Loss	*Ex: Lose 15 pounds within 6 months.*	*Ex: To feel more self-confident and project that to my family.*	
Improve Strength	*Ex: Be able to do 10 pull-ups and 20 pushups in one sitting within 3 months.*	*Ex: To go on a rock-climbing trip with friends next spring*	
Improve Muscle Tone	*Ex: Lose 5 inches around my waist and see flat abs when I stand naked in front of the mirror.*	*Ex: Decrease my risk for heart disease and diabetes while increasing libido with more testosterone from muscle tone.*	
Manage Autoimmune Flare-Ups	*Ex: Keep my eczema from coming back*	*Ex: The itchiness and irritation is really frustrating.*	
Prevent Chronic Disease	*Ex: Avoid the diabetes that has plagued my parents.*	*Ex: To not burden my children and spouse, and to have more time and energy to spend with them.*	
Stay Fit Over the Long-Term	*Ex: Maintain a size 6–8 and be able to walk 5 miles without pain until I'm in my eighties.*	*Ex: To feel comfortable in my own skin and be able to enjoy time with children and grandchildren.*	
Choose Your Own Goal			

Weight Loss

This may seem like a vast topic. In fact, I bet many of you have read multiple lengthy books just on this goal alone. While it may seem like the number-one goal that most people haver-elated to health, I would argue that weight loss is actually just an added benefit of making changes to your lifestyle and wellness choices. Dropping excess pounds is truly a wonderful side effect of being on the right path to owning your wellness.

I do not mean to minimize this, especially if it is your number-one goal. Just keep in mind that if you are already employing the nourishing strategies I have laid out above, you are likely well on the road to achieving your weight loss goals. That said, here are a few other tips and tricks I have picked up over the years that have reaped wonderful results for my clients:

Don't drink your calories. To explain this one simple rule, I'm going to go at it backward. Do you know what I tell clients who desperately need to gain weight? "Drink your calories." Why? Because the digestive system and your satiety hormones do not register calories that you consume without chewing the same way. This is why you can easily down hundreds of calories in the form of soda or juice and still have the same size meal. So when ultra-thin people need to gain, this is my go-to way to sneak pounds onto people's frames.

If weight loss is your goal, you want your body to be aware and register every nourishing calorie you take in. If you are into juicing and making smoothies, you might want to put that on the back burner for now. Think about all the ingredients you throw into your blender to make that smoothie. If you forced yourself to sit down and eat every ingredient individually, you would probably be too full and bored of eating to get it all down. Yet somehow, those same calories just fly down your throat when whipped up together!

Make sure each bite of food has nourishing qualities. Said in layman's terms: avoid empty calories. Empty calories refer to foods (or manmade foodlike items) that are lacking in vitamins, minerals, proteins, fats, and fiber. An easy

If weight loss is your goal, you want your body to be aware and register every nourishing calorie you take in.

example is a 12-ounce can of soda versus the same calories in steamed broccoli. You'd probably need about 4 or 5 cups of steamed broccoli to match the caloric equivalent of a can of soda. That's like taking a mixing bowl full of broccoli and eating every last bite. Can you imagine how gross you'd be feeling after about half of that? Not to mention the fact that you'd have no chance of wanting to eat a full meal with it. And yet, if you had sipped on the soda while having a full meal of maybe a burger and fries, that soda would not slow you down at all!

That is an easy example, but most of you already know that drinking soda is a bad idea for so many reasons. Where a lot of people get confused is with things that seem like healthy choices but really aren't supporting their goal of losing weight. My favorite example is the much-coveted breakfast staple: oatmeal. I can't tell you how many people I've had to plead with to give this one up. "But why?" they ask me. "I love my morning oatmeal; it's filling and delicious and loaded with fiber." Whether it is steel cut, slow-cooker Irish oats, or the pre-packed stuff you simply pour hot water on, oats are NOT your friend when it comes to losing weight. Sure, it seems healthy, but that stuff only turns into sugar once you've digested it. The only difference between the higher-quality oats and processed stuff is how fast it turns to sugar in your system. The fiber will slow down the digestive process, so yes, you'll stay full for an hour or so. But you are still going to get a sugar crash once it is out of your system, and you'll find yourself craving more!

Again, if I have a client wanting to gain weight, oatmeal seems like a great idea for breakfast because it will help them stay hungry all day long. That does not seem like a good plan when weight loss is what you are trying to achieve. You want food that not only burns slowly but also gives you all the things you need to thrive: proteins to help get your cortisol revving and body pumping, fats to feed the brain and help you absorb minerals and vitamins, and lots of health-promoting antioxidants and other micronutrients. A better choice might be a bowl of yogurt (non-dairy if you prefer) with some slivered almonds and a handful of berries with cinnamon on top. Or maybe some pastured eggs with a side of avocado, a drizzle of sea salt and balsamic, and some wilted greens sauteed in olive oil.

Fat will not make you fat. This little-known fact is a topic I could go on and on about, but I will do my best to make this brief. I wish desperately that there was another word for the fat on our bellies versus the fat found in food. One does not beget the other. Remember our earlier conversation on how the eighties and nineties trends of eating low- and no-fat food replacements coincided with the explosion of the obesity epidemic? If you are trying to lose weight by eating food that is not nourishing, reduced calories, and reduced fat, you are going to be hungry all day and will find yourself with nutrient deficiencies galore. This will leave you constantly yearning for another bite, a little goodie, and riding a blood sugar roller coaster all day long.

The breakfast alternatives I suggested above are not low-fat, but they are loaded with the nutrients you need to get the day going. There will be no blood sugar crash at 10 a.m. You'll be able to go straight through until lunch without having to worry about snacks. And even though calorically they are higher, the staying power they give you means you are avoiding the nibbles throughout the day.

I'm not suggesting that you "go keto." That high-fat diet craze has merit, but it has been commandeered by marketers and the meaning has been lost along the way. A truly therapeutic ketogenic diet entails fasting protocols (more on this later) combined with a diet of over 80 percent fat to manage conditions like seizures. All I'm suggesting is that you do not avoid fats in your diet. Reach for natural fats that humans have used for centuries: butter, lard, tallow, avocados, nuts, coconut, olives, and so on. These demonized foods are loaded with nourishment that will stay with you for hours and hours. Unless you have a genetic predisposition not to be able to tolerate fats, especially saturated fats, these delicious foods should definitely be part of your diet.

The only time that natural fats in the diet are going to detract from your health is when you combine them with sugar. If you think about it, there are no foods in nature that have a large amount of fat combined with sugar. Avocados are mostly fat and fiber; nuts are fat and protein. They don't go hand-in-hand in nature because we are not meant to have high doses of sugar with fat. When you combine the two, you end up with something so delicious that you can't stop eating it! The sugar overrides the satiety factor of the fat. There is a simultaneous increase in inflammation and a shutting down of hunger-regulating hormones. Fat + Sugar is truly a recipe for disaster. So if you are ready to start adding fats back into your diet, please make sure to cut back sources of sugar at the same time.

Calorie counting is passé. I'd like to address the long-held belief that calorie counting is the end-all-be-all. Calories truly matter only when they are way too low or way too high. Everything in the middle is really just about the same. If you are gaining weight, you are likely taking in too many calories for your activity, and if you're too thin and staying that way or losing more, you need

Don't focus on restriction; focus on nourishment.

more calories. What matters is that you focus on the quality of those calories, not the number! Like I've been saying all along, **nourish** yourself with what you need to thrive. ***Don't focus on restriction; focus on nourishment.***

This was not a lesson easily learned for me either. I spent most of my adolescence and young adulthood counting every morsel that crossed my lips. I'd lose brain cells counting and recounting what I'd had and what I had left to eat each day. I swear, I might have been CEO of a Fortune 500 company if I'd stopped counting calories and actually given my brain what it needed to thrive and grow. Yeesh! And once it's ingrained into you to count calories, it becomes really hard to stop. I can shovel some avocado onto my plate and know within probably five calories how much I had. So for me, switching that mindset from quantity to quality was NOT easy.

Macronutrient cycling is an alternative to calorie counting. As I moved away from counting calories, my OCD brain still wanted to have control over what I was eating. One strategy that not only filled my need for doing math all day but is quite helpful in both weight-loss/fat-loss and overall health is something called "macronutrient cycling." The term "macronutrients" refers to fat, protein, and carbohydrates. Micronutrients are things like vitamins and minerals, but with macronutrients, we are looking at the big picture of what your diet consists of. When I get people to play around with changing up their macronutrients every month or even season, they quickly get results. This can be a good strategy to employ both at the onset of weight loss and when you start hitting a plateau before you've reached your goal. I even use macro cycling to help me maintain my fitness.

When combined with changes in how you exercise, changes in your diet from one way to another kind of surprise your metabolism. Suddenly it needs new enzymes for digestion, has new sources of energy, and even gives you different outputs. When using macronutrient cycling after hitting a fitness plateau, I usually start clients with a month or two of high-protein combined with regular resistance training with relatively high reps and some interval training. Then we move to high-fat and do more work with heavy strength training and long endurance cardio. Finally, we go to more moderate ratios of fat/protein/carbs and just focus on recovery work like yoga and light-to-moderate cardio. Then we do it all over again.

These constant switches will keep their bodies from staying on the plateau or even from regressing to weight gain again. But we can use the same idea when trying to keep our body fit and constantly evolving throughout our lifetime.

As you learned above, the only constant is change, and so it should be for your diet. I suggest most people cycle through four different phases of macronutrient ratios. This can be done seasonally, monthly, or even in shorter cycles. I find that for weight/fat loss, cycles of about ten days or so are best. For people who are already at a weight and fitness level they like, longer cycles of a month or even a season are more effective. Here is an example of how I'd have someone cycle nutrients based on the seasons:

Winter: Higher carbs—40–50% carbs, 20–30% protein, 20–30% fat

Spring: Higher protein—20% carbs, 30–40% protein, 40–50% fat

Summer: Moderate ratios—30–40% carbs, 30–40% protein, 20–30% fat

Fall: Higher fat—10–20% carbs, 20–30% protein, 50–70% fat

During the winter months, many of us crave warming foods and starches like winter squashes and holiday goodies. When spring comes, we need to start shedding that winter coat and eating lighter. During summer we get to enjoy all the beautiful fruits and vegetables and are generally more active, so we need a little bit of everything. Then in the fall, we can start getting warm and cozy and increase the fat in the

85

diet. Obviously, there can be some variability within those numbers above, but the sheer act of having to find foods to eat that fit into those ratios will force you to change your diet. That means you are getting all kinds of different micronutrients in addition to macronutrients. That variety will help keep your metabolism resilient and strong.

Some people, myself included, do not do so well with the higher carbohydrate phase of this cycling plan. For me, I get too hungry and it gets me thinking about food too often, which triggers my old disordered eating brain. So if you'd prefer to take out the higher carb phase, you would instead break your cycles into just three: higher protein, moderate ratios, and higher fat. I encourage you to play around with each of these and see which order of each cycle, and for how long, works best. I like doing longer, almost seasonal cycles because it gives me a chance to get into a routine and know what kind of groceries and recipes to incorporate. But if you are more easily adapted to big changes, shorter cycles might be perfect for you.

There are many ways you can incorporate this idea into your life. I have some clients who are younger women still having regular periods cycle macros throughout the month: high fat the first ten days, higher protein the next ten, then finishing with higher carb the last ten. This helps them support their bodies' needs during each phase of their cycle. As I said earlier, some people can use macronutrient changes to shock their bodies into dropping more fat. Ladies, if you fall into this category of still cycling but want to get into fasting and macronutrient cycling, please check out Dr. Mindy Pelz at www.drmindypelz.com and Kayla Osterhoff, MPH, PhD at www.biocurious.com for a wealth of knowledge on the topic.

If you are interested in trying this strategy, I highly recommend using a good food-tracking app to do so. It takes a lot off your plate and allows you to quickly see what macros you have eaten throughout the day. I prefer Cronometer myself. I have a pro account with them that allows me to peek in on my clients' progress anytime I want to. The hardest part of using these apps is just getting into the routine of it. Once you have the basics down, it gets easier to enter recipes and whatnot. Other good options include LoseIt, Fooducate, and MyFitnessPal. A quick internet search will give you plenty of options. The one thing I caution you on here is that you don't get too bogged down in the calorie counting side of the equation and focus more on the quality of your food, not just quantity.

And ... remember all that we have discussed before:

- If you're not hungry, don't eat!
- Don't snack.
- Eat only what you love.
- Eat complete meals and get full.
- Sit down to a full plate.
- Step away from the kitchen when you're done.

Improve Strength

It bums me out that this goal is not a higher priority for most people. I can't think of any reason why you wouldn't want to be stronger. Whether you are an eighty-year-old woman who would just like to be able to carry a sack of groceries without help or a twenty-year-old man wanting to be able to pick up his girlfriend (or boyfriend) without grunting, strength is a great goal. One of my favorite new hashtag trends on social media is #strongissexy or #strongisthenewskinny. I *love* this! I needed this when I was a young teen striving to be anything but what my body was giving me. Now that I'm in my midforties, I take great pride in the strength my slight frame has.

I will discuss this specific goal more in-depth during the "Move" chapter of this book. But nothing you are going to do to improve strength is going to stick if you aren't nourishing yourself with what you need to keep that strength. Being strong doesn't just require protein; it requires some carbohydrates too. If you are trying to get strong, going super low-carb or ketogenic is probably not going to help you. If you are working on exercises and habits to consistently gain strength, you'll want to make sure your meals (pre- and post-workout) have a good ratio of healthy carbs involved. This means having some frozen berries and even some mango in a protein smoothie before a workout. This means adding a little potato or rice to accompany your dinner. This is not a license to ill when it comes to carbs. Don't go "refueling" on Yoohoo and Doritos. Reach for real food loaded with nutrients, as we've discussed all along.

And please do not worry about the old dogma that you need to get protein within thirty minutes after working out to keep the muscle you worked on. If that were true, prehistoric humans would have been spindly little runts. What matters is that you are not letting yourself go hungry. This is one of the few goals where I don't suggest you work out on a completely empty stomach (i.e., first thing in the morning). Instead, get a good breakfast in, make sure you've fully digested, then give it your all in the gym. When you are ready, refuel with a well-balanced meal.

Improve Muscle Tone

Gaining strength and improving muscle tone may seem like one and the same goal, but you'd be mistaken. If you've ever paid attention to the physiques in strong-man competitions, you know that they are not exactly well-defined. And unlike Arnold Schwarzenegger, most bodybuilders are not always all that strong. These are different goals and require different fueling strategies.

While we focus more on well-rounded meals with carbo-hydrates, fats, and protein, with an emphasis on gaining strength, we have to switch it up a bit when it comes to muscle tone. If your carbohydrate intake is too high, you may find that your muscles are hiding under a little layer of bloat. If improving the look of your muscles matters, we sure don't want to have them buried under a winter coat. Also, please know that it is okay to just want to be more toned. There is no shame in caring about how you look. If having arms that don't jiggle, or a tummy that doesn't pooch is a priority, then go get it!

Just like the strength goal, I'll give you strategies to achieve muscle tone in the "Move" chapter of this book. As you work on that, remember that you'll want to be paying attention to the timing of your meals as well as the composition. This is because eliminating excess fat and water weight will have to go hand in hand with laying down a little muscle. I highly recommend that people work out in a fasted state for this goal. That means making sure you had a well-balanced dinner: healthy fats, protein, vegetables galore, and a little starch. Get a good night's sleep. Wake up and drink your water. Then hit your workout. (Again, details to come.) You will be tapping into your fat stores for energy. Since you're rehydrated, your body won't hold onto water. Give it your all in that workout and leave sweaty. Then eat like a king!

After that fasted workout, you'll want to make sure your first meal has plenty of protein. This is a meal where you might want a little more protein than you'd normally have. If you don't enjoy eating eggs, bacon, and so on, you might want to make yourself a smoothie (not a juice) that is loaded with high-quality protein. I suggest that people reach for collagen protein and either a plant-based protein powder (that is primarily hemp and/or pea protein) or a whey protein powder (if you tolerate dairy). Then get lots of colorful produce involved: avocados, berries, greens, and so on. Finally, drizzle your meal or smoothie with satisfying fats that add tons of flavor: coconut/oil, nuts, avocados, and so on. This morning meal needs to help your body recover from your workout effectively and keep you going for many hours to come. As you let your body recover and rest, you'll find you start to see that muscle tone appear very quickly.

Manage Autoimmune Flare-Ups

Autoimmunity is a very broad term that refers to your body's immune system essentially getting confused and attacking itself. Autoimmunity flare-ups can manifest in many ways, some of which are quite subtle. Examples are eczema, psoriasis, chronic allergies or sinus congestion, achy joints, foggy thinking, unexplained headaches, dry eyes, and the list goes on and on. Autoimmunity is at the base of many chronic issues we deal with in modern society: arthritis, irritable bowel, chronic fatigue, thyroid disorders, dermatitis, and seasonal allergies. There may even be an autoimmune element to osteoporosis, Alzheimer's and dementia, diabetes, and multiple sclerosis. Unfortunately, due to the modern lifestyle of chronic stress, processed foods, lack of time in nature, and exposure to toxins, many people struggle with some form of autoimmunity. If any of the above symptoms or diagnoses sound familiar to you and/or your loved ones, then you might want to pay a little attention to this section.

When the immune system is either overloaded or confused, we have to work to help it out. One way we can calm down a flare-up of autoimmunity is to not burden the immune system with things that are known to be taxing on it. When it comes to nutrition, this means eliminating some of the most likely offenders (foods that are common allergens). These include cow's dairy, eggs, nightshades, nuts, seeds, alcohol, gluten, and most grains. And as daunting as all those seem to eliminate, they are not nearly a complete list. During the "Explore" chapter of this book, I will help you find ways to figure out which foods might be triggers for you. I will also show you how to try your own elimination diet and, more importantly, how to try to reintroduce foods into your life. If you know that autoimmune issues are at the base of your main health complaints and are holding you back from your goals, you should definitely dig deeper into the "Explore" chapter to help you find out why and what is triggering you. For more advanced reading on the topic of following a strict autoimmune protocol, I highly recommend the book *A Simple Guide to the Paleo Autoimmune Protocol* by Eileen Laird.

The Paleo diet is one of the simplest formats to follow when first attempting to manage conditions you suspect might be related to autoimmunity. The Paleo diet at its core excludes grains, dairy, refined sugars, artificial/processed foods, legumes, and all processed oils. When I first heard about Paleo over a decade ago, I started reading everything I could get my hands on. Within a couple of weeks of starting this plan, I was not only leaning out but suddenly wasn't getting the scaly patches of eczema on my shoulders and belly. My chronic achiness under my kneecaps and in my rotator cuffs just disappeared. It sounds ridiculous, but I was in shock at how quickly it worked! I don't think that everyone should eat the Paleo diet, but if you are trying to deal with any of the issues discussed in this section, it sure won't hurt. Here are some good resources to get you started if you're interested:

- *The Paleo Solution: The Original Human Diet* by Robb Wolf

- *The Paleo Approach: Reverse Autoimmune Disease and Heal Your Body* by Sarah Ballantyne

- *Practical Paleo* by Diane Sanfilippo

- *The Primal Blueprint* by Mark Sisson

I'm certainly not suggesting that everyone go on a Paleo diet. However, if you know that autoimmune issues are something that you contend with, the Paleo template is a very good way to get started in the right direction. Once you have found ways to eliminate some of the more triggering foods from your diet, you'll then be ready to layer in major nourishment. For my clients who are dealing with conditions like multiple sclerosis or rheumatoid arthritis, I highly recommend they start following the "Wahls Protocol." I learned about Dr. Terry Wahls many years ago when I was first getting into the Paleo movement. As hard as it may seem to believe, she has reversed her very debilitating MS by finding all the micronutrients she needs from a very strategic and whole foods–based diet. She took the Paleo idea and then ramped it up to the next level to figure out just how much of what nutrients you need from which foods to maximize your nutrient intake to manage autoimmunity. If this sounds interesting to you, I suggest you pick up a copy of *The Wahls Protocol*. It is an autoimmune game-changer!

Prevent Chronic Disease

Doesn't that sound like a simple concept? And yet how on earth does one go about doing so? Again, I need to remind you that I do not claim to prevent or treat any disease. However, I can surely give you some great ways to at least try to avoid some of the big ones. If you have specific chronic diseases that run in your family, you will want to be a little extra cautious not to increase your chances of having to contend with them later on. If you don't know about your genetic propensities, I recommend doing a little digging with some DNA testing. More on this type of testing and how to utilize it in our "Explore" chapter. However, many of us need to work to prevent diseases just based on how prevalent they are in our modern society. Here are some of the big ones and some simple strategies to employ to try to stave off these all-too-common chronic diseases:

Diabetes: By this, I mean type 2 diabetes, which is brought on by lifestyle and dietary choices. Our bodies are designed to handle only so much sugar (and things that turn into sugar once digested) at once. When you consume levels of carbohydrates that are too high for your specific chemistry and do so over a long period, you will likely end up with pre-diabetes and eventually full-blown diabetes if you aren't changing your ways. This is where you need to figure out what level of carbohydrate intake is appropriate for YOU!

There are simple ways to tell if you are not having the right amount of carbs. Symptoms of blood sugar dysregulation include

- carrying more than twenty to thirty pounds of extra weight.
- feeling like you cannot go without food for more than a few hours.
- carrying your extra weight around your midsection.
- craving sweets regularly.
- foggy thinking.

The list goes on and on, but to keep it simple, if you think you are eating too many carbohydrates for your personal chemistry, you probably are. The easiest way to get started on bringing your intake into a more healthy range is just to get rid of all empty carbohydrate foods. This includes things like bread, pasta, crackers, cereal, rice, and of course cookies, juice, and most desserts. You don't have to adopt a low-carb diet in order to combat diabetes. You just need to make sure that every carbohydrate you take in is nutritious, has plenty of fiber, and adds to your health instead of taking away from it.

For most people, just swapping out bread and pasta for vegetables will make all the difference in the world for their blood sugars. Again, I do not claim to cure disease, but I have had many clients over the years come to me after their doctor said they were "pre-diabetic" and needed to fix things fast. The fear of having to be on insulin or to deal with all the long-term detrimental effects of diabetes was enough to scare them into making some diet and lifestyle changes. I have watched countless clients reverse their pre-diabetic diagnosis, and many have even reversed type 2 diabetes! Below are examples of swaps I've helped my clients make that have brought down their blood sugars to the point that diabetes was no longer on the table:

- Ditching oatmeal for breakfast and replacing it with yogurt or cottage cheese with fresh berries

- Swapping morning toast for a couple of eggs and pasture-raised bacon

- Drinking a big glass of water before morning coffee, and passing on the juice

- Making sure to get full at breakfast and lunch to help avoid the breakroom pastries and other temptations

- Opting for an open-faced sandwich and ditching half the bread—or better yet, having a large salad with extra protein on top at lunch

- Making starches like potatoes a garnish to dinner and not the main event

- Focusing on making their plates at least 50 percent vegetables

- Allowing desserts in small portions and only on special occasions

- Not having any trigger foods or tempting goodies at home, which means having to leave the house to make an event of enjoying their favorite treats

None of these ideas above are earth-shattering, ground-breaking ideas. I'm not original or unique here. However, the people I gave this advice to were all dealing with some very scary alternatives. Unfortunately, when they get referred to talk to a dietician, they are often sold the old "My Plate" plan of basing most of their meals on whole grains, keeping fats to a minimum, and eating lean protein. Why is it so hard to just understand that lowering your sugar intake brings down your blood sugars? It seriously never ceases to amaze me! Just because you have family members struggling with diabetes or a doctor telling you that you are in for a lifetime of insulin injections doesn't mean you can't make changes right now. *You have control, but start today.*

You have control, but start today.

Heart disease: The topic of how to nourish yourself to prevent heart disease has become a hot-button issue as of late. You'll recall that early in this section, I talked about how our modern (last fifty years or so) government guidelines on what a healthy diet should be have been greatly misguided. Sadly, that has not changed, and doctors today are still encouraging their patients to eat high-carb and low-fat. Although the science does not support the idea that eating cholesterol and fat increases your body's cholesterol and fat, they just can't shake this dogma. I'm here to tell you—that's just flat wrong.[6]

Some people have a genetic predisposition to not metabolizing saturated fats and cholesterol well and have chronically high cholesterol (like over 300) no matter what they eat. If you are one of these people, feel free to skip this section and read more about preventing heart disease in the "Move" chapter of this book. But for the rest of us, this doesn't have to be hard. As Michael Pollan, author of *The Omnivore's Dilemma*, says, "Eat food. Not too much. Mostly plants."

Remember Dr. Nasha's "Perfect Plate"? I sure hope those two people have met because she put together the exact picture of what he was suggesting. ***Almost every dietary plan I have ever seen has just one thing in common: eat your veggies.*** With the exception of Dr. Atkins and those following the carnivore diet, few would argue that plants, plants, plants are the way to increase your health. What will certainly contribute to all diseases, heart disease included, is too much sugar, over-processed foods, and not enough veggies. You don't even have to count fat grams or calories. Just load each plate with as much produce as possible, have some healthy protein to make sure you're full, sprinkle fatty flavors, and avoid sweets.

Other chronic diseases such as dementia and cancer: All of the advice I have offered above to stave off heart disease and diabetes applies to almost all chronic ailments. Of course, there is nothing I can do to change your family history, genetics, and even your environment. By living in the modern world, we are innately exposed to a whole slew of modern-day stressors and toxins that humans are just not yet designed to cope with. Our world and technologies may have progressed, but our physiology is slower in its development. But you do have control over how you nourish yourself.

> Almost every dietary plan I have ever seen has just one thing in common: eat your veggies.

If you have a family history of dementia and dementia-related ailments, I encourage you to read some of Dr. David Perlmutter's work. When I picked up a copy of *Grain Brain* years ago, it was a complete paradigm shift for me. Well, not just me, because he's sold over a million copies to date.

The idea that Alzheimer's and dementia don't have to just "happen" to you but that you have any modicum of control was truly groundbreaking. Since then, there has been much research into the idea that overconsumption of sugar over the long term can contribute to loss of cognition. In fact, there is some evidence to suggest that dementia is a form of what is now being called type 3 diabetes!

Again, I'm not telling you that you can cure your cognitive decline by simply eating better. But—what if you could? What if a healthier diet over your lifetime could cut your chances of all kinds of chronic diseases? What if swapping juice for the actual fruit, or bread for potato was enough to stop you from causing systemic inflammation? What if just drinking more water and putting down the extra cocktail on the weekend was the difference between being a healthy nonagenarian and suffering from a stroke at seventy? What if?

I want to help you put all the health information out there into the context of *you*. ***How can you make small changes today that will have big impacts on your health over the long term?*** If you listed "prevent chronic disease_____" as

> How can you make small changes today that will have big impacts on your health over the long term?

your main health goal, then make changes today! Sure, dropping the weekly trip to Baskin Robbins may not stop you from having to fight cancer or heart disease. But what if it did? Wouldn't it be better to at least try?

Stay Fit over the Long Term

Some of you may be thinking that this doesn't seem like a reasonable goal. I would argue you are quite wrong. I know many people who didn't even achieve their peak fitness until their midfifties. In fact, I've seen many in their sixties and seventies reach a level of fitness they only thought possible in their youth. My parents are still able to hike five miles at a good clip, travel, and even compete in golf and tennis tournaments. My maternal grandparents are in their midnineties and still read avidly, do basic exercises in their community gym, and take walks around their retirement community. Now, of course, we may have some good genetics working in our favor, but they all did their best to eat well, not overindulge, and stay active.

You don't have to hit the gym five days a week to be a fit octogenarian, but you do have to focus on good basic nutrition and self-care. All of the advice I've given above to stave off chronic disease is also going to help you stay fit for decades to come. However, there is one strategy we haven't yet discussed that has a pretty good track record in helping people get in and stay in shape for decades: intermittent fasting.

If there is any diet trend that is more controversial or over-discussed, it has to be intermittent fasting (IF). Honestly, I put this term into the same category as "mindful eating" because what does it really mean? Like mindfulness, it's a fancy way of saying what you should be doing anyway. Just like we should be paying attention to what we eat, we should also occasionally *stop* eating!

Human physiology was designed way before modern refrigeration and food preservation was developed. Our bodies are not meant to be in a constant state of noshing throughout the day. Our digestion needs a break between feedings to fully process what we've eaten and move on to other physiological functions—like exercise and detoxification. Fasting is also just a way of life for humans all over the world. Almost all major religions have some form of fasting involved in their rituals. Why? Because abstaining helps a person find clarity and allows the mind and body to detoxify and start fresh.

I'm not going to dig deep into the science of IF because one quick Google search will give you so many hits your head will explode. Also, because this doesn't have to be complicated. *After you finish your last meal of the day, stop eating. That's it.* Seriously! Just stop. Make sure you've put enough time between dinner and breakfast the next day to allow your system to reset. This means you've blown through your blood sugar and liver glycogen and have started tapping into your body fat for energy to feed your brain and body. When you employ at least twelve hours between the last meal of the day and the first of the next day, you allow your body to get into "ketosis." This is a natural state of burning fat ketones for energy and not depending on sugar.

After you finish your last meal of the day, stop eating. That's it.

The "keto diet" is just a play on this basic human concept of fasting from one day to the next. Yes, many will then go on a high-fat diet to try to keep this state going, but they are just tapping into their body's innate wisdom to use its fat stores for energy. That is the whole reason humans store fat—to be able to use it when there are times of want.

I believe that *all* humans (even children) should be able to fast for twelve hours a day. Which, if you think about it, is not weird at all. If you have dinner at 7:30 p.m., that just means you don't have breakfast until 7:30 a.m. Even kids do this without thinking about it. However, if you are trying to get your body to burn more stored body fat for energy, then pushing that fast to fourteen to sixteen hours might be helpful. This means that breakfast/brunch is around 9:30–11:30 a.m. That's all. Seriously not a big deal. Many of us do this on the weekends just by mistake.

The most important thing to keep in mind when fasting is that the real magic happens in how you "break-the-fast." Breakfast is only the most important meal of the day because you turn off the fasting mechanism. If you wake up

The most important thing to keep in mind when fasting is that the real magic happens in how you "break-the-fast."

and are in a ketogenic fat-burning state, wouldn't you want to keep that going as long as possible? Yes! So don't break the fast with sugar/starch. That first meal should be high in protein, fats, and fibrous produce to keep you from switching all the way back to sugar-burning. Things like eggs, yogurt, bacon, avocado, berries, and cottage cheese are all great options for getting your day started strong and keeping you lean!

One note of caution: If you are a woman of child-bearing years (meaning you still have your period), do not try to push the fasting beyond fourteen hours or so. For you, hormones rely on a sufficient nutrient intake to stay fertile and keep you cycling regularly. If you are in this category, I highly recommend watching some of the awesome videos on YouTube by Dr. Mindy Pelz, or checking out her latest book, *Fast like a Girl*. Through her videos, Facebook groups, and YouTube channel, she illustrates how to utilize fasting within your cycle to maximize your results while still maintaining fertility. Her methods can also be applied to those who are menopausal.

One group of people who should definitely not try

fasting are those who are underweight (a BMI under 19) or have a history of disordered eating. Trying to add fasting beyond twelve hours may further push your weight down into a danger zone.

IF + macronutrient cycling: If you flip back to the section on weight loss under "Does It Support Your Goal?" take a look at the bit about macronutrient cycling. In particular, I delineate how to change your diet based on the seasons. When you combine this principle with intermittent fasting, I believe you will have a recipe for owning your wellness for the rest of your life!

Go Back to Your Goal Setting

Now that you have read through various strategies to help you reach your goal(s), please flip back to the chart you filled out at the beginning of this section. Look at the areas you filled out: General Goal, Specific Goal, Why, and Personal Notes. If any of your original thoughts around that goal have changed since reading through this section, please take time now to erase them and start over. Once you are happy with what you've written, it is time to start putting some plans into place to finally reach that goal.

For each goal that you decide to focus on, please write down at least one way you will utilize what you've learned in the "Nourish" chapter of this book. You may find it easier to even break that action down into smaller stages. Below you'll

see a place to write down your plan of action next to each of
your goals. Again, I've given you an example to guide you.
Please don't gloss over this section. You've done a great job
already figuring out what you want to achieve and why. Now
we will start working on the *how*.

Specific Goal	Why?	Action Item 1	Action Item 2	Action Item 3
Ex: Stay healthy over the long term	*To be able to play with my grandchildren and travel in retirement*	*Rotate macros by season*	*Stretch out daily fasts to 14 hours/day*	*Eat only when hungry*

Mapping Out Your Days

I hope that you are not feeling overwhelmed with mapping out how to reach your goals. This might be a good time for us to just talk about some basics to help you as you continue on those action items you just lined up for yourself.

Regardless of your specific goal, many of us just want to eat healthier and feel good every day. Below are some very simple strategies I use to help most of my health coaching clients get going on the right path. And we have to start with the most important meal of the day.

Breakfast

To expound a bit on what we already touched on with intermittent fasting, let's revisit breaking the fast. Remember, breakfast matters because you are "breaking the fast." That's actually where the word comes from. Most of us finished eating a couple of hours before bedtime. By the time we are drifting into a deep sleep, we have hopefully blown through most of our blood sugar and are starting to tap into our liver glycogen and, eventually, body fat stores for energy. So by the time we wake in the morning, we are fat-burning machines! Once you have switched to burning fat for energy, the end product is ketones. These can be used to fuel our bodies and minds when there is no more sugar to be processed. You are literally breaking down your muffin tops and saddlebags for energy.

The last thing you want to do first thing in the morning is switch your metaolism right back to burning sugar for energy.

The last thing you want to do first thing in the morning is switch your metabolism right back to burning sugar for energy. This is actually the time you want to try to use that fat metabolism to your benefit. First, you should start each morning with a tall glass of water. Aside from not having food for many hours, you have also been dehydrated. So take this time to drink a big glass of water (8–16 oz.) before you even leave your bathroom in the morning. I make sure to take a glass with me at night before I go to bed and finish it off before I leave the bedroom to start my day. Full disclosure, I have borrowed this idea of a morning "inner bath" from the amazing Shawn Stevenson of *The Model Health* podcast.[7]

Once you've had your "inner bath" and rehydrated, you might consider a workout if your schedule allows it. Whether you're in the mood for gentle yoga, a long walk, or a high-intensity boot camp, it really doesn't matter. As long as you get your body moving, you'll continue using your body's fat stores for energy. Just don't forget the water, because dehydration will make you feel like you're hungry even when your body would be just fine using its own fat for energy. Don't fall prey to thinking you can't work out without eating first; it's just not true. You can, and you'll see faster gains in your fitness by doing so.

Even if you don't have time for a workout but need to get to a meeting or whatever is in your day, just try to see if you can push breaking the fast out a bit longer. You'll be surprised at how a little water and maybe some caffeine can help you get things done with laser-sharp thinking when your brain is using ketones for energy instead of a pastry. This is actually where the whole "bulletproof coffee" idea came from. This high-fat/caffeine combo was popularized by Dave Asprey in the early 2000s because he realized that by allowing his body and brain to run on ketones for energy instead of switching back to sugar-burning, he was able to stay fasted longer and be more efficient and effective.

But eventually, you will need to break the fast, and that's when it's critical you have a good strategy. Unless you are severely underweight, most everyone would do well to start their day with a high-fat, high-protein, and low-carbohydrate breakfast. This will not only help you to keep burning a little fat for energy but the added protein will help your body's natural cortisol rhythm. In the morning, we want our cortisol (natural stress hormone) to peak, and having a little protein will help that in the morning. Think of it this way: you know how when you're super stressed or worn out in the evening you get a craving for something sugary/starchy/yummy? That's because you want some carbs to help feed into your serotonin (calming hormone) and get you into a cozy mood. That's the last thing we need first thing in the morning!

Even if you don't have any desire to lose weight, focusing on having a high-protein, high-fat, low-carb breakfast will help you start the day strong. Here are a few examples of breakfast ideas that you might try incorporating into your day:

- Eggs and leftover veggies from last night's dinner. I like serving this over a cauliflower-based crepe (Crepini is a preferred brand in my house).

- Pastured bacon or sausage with a bowl of seasonal organic berries with some coconut cream drizzled over the top.

- Unsweetened yogurt (dairy, coconut, or nut-based) loaded with chopped nuts, organic berries, and shaved coconut flakes.

- Frittatas are a great way to use up eggs and veggies that need to be eaten. You can whip them together, with or without a little cheese, and bake in muffin tins for an easy breakfast anytime. These are great with a side of sliced avocado and a sprinkle of sea salt.

Hopefully, you get the idea. Even if none of the above sounds appealing to you, think about things you enjoy eating that are low in carbohydrates and high in protein and fat. You'll notice I mentioned things like berries and avocado in there. That's because these fruits are inherently very low in carbohydrates and high in fiber. If you've been the kind of person that has to put a banana in your smoothie or just loves bananas on yogurt, try swapping it out for avocado or berries. And for those of you who eat your banana every day for the potassium, please know that half an avocado has about 65 mg more potassium than a medium banana.[8]

When I first start working with a client, breaking the fast is usually one of our first projects. If you just focus on this one change, I think you'll find it sets you up for making better decisions the rest of the day.

Lunch

This brings us to lunch. I like to use the metaphor of a keystone for the meal in the middle of the day. Think about an arched doorway lined with big stones. My mind immediately goes to every castle in *Game of Thrones*. Anyway, those stones all stack up to a central keystone. This usually broader and stronger stone must be placed just right to keep the integrity of the doorway. If this stone is removed, the whole thing collapses.

Lunch needs to be your keystone. If you get just the right mix of nutrients and fullness here, you'll be successful the rest of the day. When clients complain to me that they need to work on what they are eating, it usually involves some version of it all falling apart in the afternoon. They have a light lunch or just snack their way through lunch and are left feeling peckish within an hour or two. Then they reach for a snack or two, and maybe do a little grazing until they start planning dinner. They feel bad about not eating well earlier, so dinner is too light, and then they are nibbling again before bed. Sound vaguely familiar?

Well, if you make lunch your keystone, the integrity of that doorway (morning on one side, afternoon on the other) ends up being strong and steady. Assuming you started the day by breaking the fast with good choices, you'll likely make it to lunch without needing a snack. When you get there, it is critically important that you make a *meal*. Not a series of small snacks. Not half a salad or half a sandwich because you're really not hungry. No. A *meal*. Remember, it's okay to eat and get full. Because when you give your tummy a full meal to feel satisfied and work on digesting, you will be able to go for many hours without needing any other snacks.

I know that many of you are arguing right now that if you eat a full meal at lunch, you'll be so full that you will need a nap and not be able to work or think straight in the afternoon. What is the alternative? Not feeling full or satisfied, then having to interrupt your workday multiple times so you can nosh on yet another goodie to keep you going? What if you taught yourself to have a solid lunch and just get back to the grind (whatever your afternoon grind may be)?

My guess—no—what I know, is that after several days, you'd find you enjoy having a nice solid meal for lunch. You'd learn that it feels good to not be thinking about food all afternoon and to enjoy the productivity that comes with that freed-up brain space!

Lunch should be a well-rounded combination of all the macronutrients. A good portion of protein, some healthy fats for taste, and plenty of veggies (maybe with a little starch). I say "a little starch" because too much comfort food in the middle of the day is going to make you want to lie down. You want food that is nourishing, not too energizing, and not too sedating either. Here are a few examples of a balanced lunch:

- A large salad with at least 4 ounces of protein, some cut-up fresh veggies, some sprinkles of cheese or olives for fat and flavor, a combination of spices you enjoy, and a healthy pour of olive oil and vinegar or some other dressing (not low-fat).

- A boxed lunch with various goodies similar to a crudités/charcuterie platter: sliced cheese, fresh-cut veggies like carrots, snow peas, bell pepper, celery, and cucumber, and a handful of nuts, a quarter cup of hummus or similar, and sliced proteins like salami, prosciutto, and so on.

- Deconstructed taco plate: two small corn tortillas loaded with tender meat like carne asada or carnitas, shredded lettuce, fajita veggies (sauteed in olive oil), some shredded cheese, and half a sliced avocado.

I bet quite a few of you thought: "There's no way I could eat all that in the middle of the day!" Not true. You probably already do. It's just that you do it in smaller nibbles and never register true hunger followed by fullness. Just try this for a few days and see how it frees you up the rest of the afternoon into the evening. Notice that while all the above meals seem really filling, none of them are high in starch. Moderate, yes, but not high. This is because we want to save that for the last meal of the day: dinner.

Dinner

A brief note here before I get too detailed on the dinner thing. There is a reason that I don't put a "snack" in between lunch and dinner (or breakfast and lunch for that matter). If you are eating a satisfying meal, you will not need one. You certainly won't need multiple snacks throughout the day. You should break the fast with a low-carbohydrate but nutrient-dense meal. Then, when you get around to lunch, you should eat a well-balanced and filling meal there too. Sure, you might get a hunger pang here and there in the late afternoon or early evening, but nothing you can't quell with a little water and activity.

By the time you get to dinner, you should be hungry. No, like legit hungry! Remember, it's okay to get hungry. It will make that meal so much more satisfying if you are really ready for it. Just about the time you're starting to think about food again in the late afternoon/early evening is when you should make a plan for dinner. What will the main course be? What sides sound good? Where will you eat it? Who with? Maybe it's a chill night at home alone. In which case, you can put on some good music and set the table for one. Maybe it's a chaotic night with multiple kids and family members. In that case, buckle up and enjoy the ride. Whatever the dinner situation

"If you fail to plan, you plan to fail."

is, you need to plan. Ben Franklin wasn't talking about meal planning, but his adage sure rings true, *"If you fail to plan, you plan to fail."*

Once you know the plan, all you have to do is execute, enjoy, and clean up. Dinner is a really good time to get back to the basics of mindful eating as we discussed earlier. Whether at home alone or out to dinner, make it an experience. It should be delicious and enjoyable. Again, you want to eat enough at this meal to feel like you are *done* eating for the day. While you don't need to be stuffed, you need to be full enough not to end up back in the kitchen again later. That is one of the many reasons that I encourage clients to put a little starch in their dinner meals. A little rice, potato, or even bread can help you kill the cravings for carbs late at night.

There's a reason we crave "comfort foods" at night. They are generally high in simple carbohydrates, which feed into serotonin (our calming hormone). Serotonin helps feed into melatonin, which is a hormone that helps us get to sleep. At dinner, we want the opposite effect of breakfast: we want to chill out after. That doesn't mean you should be eating mac and cheese for dinner, but it means you should definitely give yourself some wiggle room on the carbs here. I'd much rather hear that you enjoyed a little sweet potato magic with your roast and veggies than know that you were raiding the cookie bin before bed. *Kill the cravings before they start.*

> ## Kill the cravings before they start.

All that said, we also need sufficient protein at dinner to keep hunger from striking in the middle of the night. Many of you don't have this problem, but some do. Middle-of-the-night eating is a sign of many detrimental clues to your health. If you're waking in the wee hours and ready to nosh, it tells me (a) dinner was insufficient or too early, (b) you are struggling with blood sugar dysregulation, and (c) there are issues with your stress hormones that are not allowing you to get a good night's sleep. Most likely, you are dealing with a combination of all the above. The best way to combat this middle-of-the-night eating issue is to get some good slow-burning protein and fats into dinner and top them off with a little starch. By making sure that your evening protein portion is significant (enough to get you full), you will find that it burns through you slowly overnight and allows you to get a good night's sleep free of snacks.

Here are a couple of examples of dinner meals that are nourishing but also help you get to bed without snacking:

- A hearty bowl of bone broth-based soup or stew with copious veggies (potatoes, carrots, leeks, mushrooms, etc.), and protein like beef or shredded chicken. For added fats, maybe a side salad with a dollop of your favorite dressing (homemade, preferably) and sliced avocado on top.

- My simple eating-out formula of lean protein*, a large side of veggies with olive oil or drawn butter on top, and small portions of starch like roasted potatoes or rice. My husband likes to go out for steak often, and I find that steak houses have the *best* veggie sides.

*The only time I worry about whether or not my protein is low-fat is when I'm at a restaurant where the quality of the meat/fish/poultry is questionable. If, for some reason, the animal was raised in a not-so-great environment and being fed not-so-great food itself, the toxins (antibiotics, pesticides, etc.) are more likely to be found in the fat of the animal. When you only eat the protein, you are at least lowering your toxic burden. All that said, please take the time to find restaurants that purchase their proteins from local and reputable sources.

As you start to find some go-to recipes that work for you and your family, you'll want to expand your planning to make grocery shopping easier. I find it helpful to make a note of which recipes I plan to make for the week and compile my grocery list on the weekend. I encourage you to cook enough of one recipe to have leftovers for at least one day. That means you aren't saddled with starting afresh every single evening. If home-cooked meals are too tedious for you to handle, find meal delivery services like HelloFresh and Hungryroot that take the work out of eating to support your goals.

Social Events

Finally, let's talk about keeping all that you've learned so far in the context of going out. You've set your goal(s), figured out your "why," and have put in place new strategies to help you eat well, feel nourished, and make progress. And then, you have a wedding to go to, or a birthday party, or a baby shower, or whatever. Life happens, and it is important that you feel like you can go out, make good decisions, enjoy the event, and still stay on the right path toward achieving your goals.

First and foremost, you need to keep in mind *why* you are at the event to begin with! You are there to celebrate something or someone. ***The celebration is the whole reason for being there. Not the food.*** Contrary to years of thinking that food is love, food is happiness, food is family, we are wrong. The joy in each event comes from the celebration: the coming together to honor something or someone. Focus on the conversations, on enjoying the company of people you maybe haven't seen in a while. While a lot of time and energy likely went into the food planning and preparation for said event, it is still not the only reason you are there. Keep that in mind as you plan out the rest of that experience.

The celebration is the whole reason for being there. Not the food.

Before you attend a social gathering, it's a good idea to make sure you don't walk into it already ravenous. Don't make the mistake of thinking that starving yourself all day means you can eat whatever you want at the event. That is a recipe for pain (I speak from experience on this one). If it is an evening event, make sure to get your breakfast and lunch meals in as usual. Yes, you could make them slightly lighter, but not by much. The goal is to show up with a little hunger but not be so starving that you grab at anything put in front of you!

Depending on the setup of the event, your top priority is to situate yourself so that you are not standing right next to the food all night. If it is a cocktail setup or buffet style, find a place to converse with people far enough from the food table that you have to go out of your way to grab the next bite.

I know we already discussed this, but it bears repeating: do not nibble your way through the event. If there are hors d'oeuvres being passed around, take what you like and put them all together on one cocktail plate or napkin. Try not to eat them separately, as you will never remember how much you put in your mouth. If you have several bites in front of you all on one plate, you're much more likely to physically and mentally feel fullness from those appetizers. If there is a buffet table for the meal, again, make sure to put all your food on one plate. Go to your table and take just a minute to really look at what you have put together for yourself. You'll be surprised how much more satisfied you feel when you just take that time to put your plate together instead of nibbling your way through the meal.

Do not feel guilty for not trying everything there is. This is not the last meal or event you will ever go to, so don't eat like it is. Remember, you should love everything you eat. If it doesn't taste that good, don't have any more. If there was one (or two) things that were just out-of-this-world amazing, by all means, go for seconds. Just keep in mind what you have already eaten and what might still be coming for dessert. If it is an event where you know dessert will really be "worth it," you might want to consider that when choosing the starches with your meal. Maybe hold back on bread/crackers/rice so that you can enjoy the sugary/starchy dessert option instead. You want to be able to leave the party feeling like you didn't deprive yourself, but not guilty for overindulging either. Maybe it is a birthday party, but is it your birthday party? If not, maybe a sliver of cake is enough. Are they serving some dessert that is your absolute favorite? Then you probably ought to have some. Is the dessert just blah, and you couldn't care less? Then that's an easy out for not going nuts and leaving there feeling great.

Keep alcohol in check. If you imbibe, you likely have an idea of what your personal tolerance is. *The easiest rule of thumb to use is to drink as much water as alcohol (if not more).* So for every glass of booze, you have the same ounces of water before the next cocktail. Also, think of the alcohol calories as you would starch. If you know you want to have some yummy starch with the main meal or there is a dessert you like, pick your poison. There is no reason to have the booze, the bread, and the bananas foster! If you don't drink, good on you. But keep in mind that juice and other caloric beverages also go in this category when it comes to keeping your sugar and starch load in check. Try not to drink your calories but to chew them instead.

Whatever the situation looks like around food, keep your focus on the people and the experience. If you remind yourself that you are there for the celebration of _____, you will be successful every time!

> The easiest rule of thumb to use is to drink as much water as alcohol (if not more).

Goals + Mapping Out Your Days

When we last looked at your goals, you added some action items. These were actual tools and strategies to help you start working toward your goals. Flip back to that section now, and let's think about how you can add some of the additional tips you learned in the last conversation about mapping out your days. Are there things you'd like to change in relation to how you organize breakfast, lunch, or dinner? Do you go out socially a lot and need to institute some of the tricks I outlined above? Here is a place to add those notes.

Specific Goal & Your "Why"	Previous Action Item(s)	Additional Tweaks to Map Out Your Day	Additional Changes for Eating Out and Social Events

Once you have this chart filled out, please mark this page, as we will come back and refer to it later.

Remember: The Only Constant Is CHANGE

Don't forget what we talked about earlier—you are a dynamic creature. Your body is constantly changing, your needs are forever different, and your goals will likely change as well. When you notice that your nutrition seems to not be working for you quite as well as it once did, it's time to reevaluate.

Don't get stuck in a rut. If low-carb worked for you for a year or so, great. But maybe it's time to try sprinkling in some potatoes or rice again. If you always lost weight and kept it off by

Don't get stuck in a rut.

going vegetarian, but your energy is now lagging and your muscle tone is lacking, it might be time to up the protein. Go back through this section, establish some new *why's* and goals, and then map out your days all over again. Don't get frustrated with yourself; just make the changes. Now.

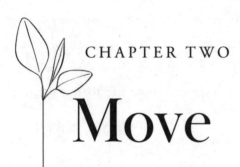

CHAPTER TWO

Move

Not everyone needs to "exercise." *Everyone, and I mean everyone, needs to move.* What is the difference? Movement is innate to the human experience and critical to our wellness. While exercising is movement, keep in mind that it is a relatively new concept. For most of our existence on this planet, humans have had to move just to survive. Now that our survival is not necessarily

Everyone, and I mean everyone, needs to move.

dependent on constant movement throughout the day, we have to "exercise."

The fact that we need to exercise to stay healthy is proof of how crucial movement is. If we still had to hunt for our food, harvest all our vegetables, tend to our children all day, and even build our own dwellings, none of us would have to get on a treadmill. Heck, if I went back in time to tell my great-grandparents in Syria that I make my living showing people how to squat, push and pull, and how to eat better so they don't get overweight, they would think I was making it up! How is it possible that in just a little over a century, we went from having a goal of finally getting to sit down at the end of a day to the goal of finally getting a "workout" in?

Nowadays, most of us really do have to get exercise because our activities of daily living are not so active. Between working from home, grocery and meal delivery, Amazon, and on-demand streaming television, we don't even have to leave our homes at all. We can literally make money, spend money, eat like a king, and have all the entertainment we ever wanted, all from the comfort of our couches. And with new virtual reality, we can even travel the world. While all of that is really remarkable and gives us so much flexibility with how we spend our time, it is not so kind to our posture and waistlines!

Why We Need to Move
(Or as Some Might Call It: "Exercise")

To put it simply, we need to exercise if we don't move enough. That's it. If you are the kind of person who gets up early and takes their dog for a walk, tends to a lovely garden during the day, meets up with friends for a hike later, and spends an hour carefully preparing a nice dinner, you probably don't need to worry about additional exercise. I think I just described my mom to a tee! But for the rest of us mortals, we probably need to fill in some gaps in our movement through the day. If the basic daily movement you engage in is not enough to maintain muscle tone,

> To put it simply, we need to exercise if we don't move enough.

keep a strong core and posture, and keep excess weight off, then it is not enough by itself. It's that simple.

Now we go back to your goals and your "why" from the "Nourish" chapter to help guide you through this next chapter regarding movement. Before you read through the rest of this, please flip back to the last page in the "Nourish" chapter and copy below your goals and *why's*. Then, take a moment to think about all the activities you do during the week. Your list doesn't have to be perfect, but to the best of your ability, write down all the activities you do and how (if at all) you think that movement supports attaining your goal(s).

Goal	Why

Own Your Wellness

Day of the Week	Movement Activity	How It Supports Your Goal
Monday	*Ex: Afternoon hike with friends*	*Ex: Gets my heart pumping and is a long caloric burn that is still fun and gets me out of the house.*
Tuesday		
Wednesday		
Thursday		
Friday		
Saturday		
Sunday		

If it wasn't easy for you to put down some sort of activity you're currently doing every day of the week, then we have work to do. Again, you do not need to exercise every day, but you really need to move! Think about how much better you feel when you take a little walk around the block to clear your head. How good does it feel to stand up from your desk and stretch out your back? Isn't it great how energized you feel after playing with kids in the park? Or joining friends for a game of tennis or golf? How can we incorporate things like this into our daily life? And on the days where movement doesn't naturally fit in, let's incorporate an exercise plan to keep you moving.

Don't Do It If You Don't Like It

I spend a lot of time with clients talking about what type of exercise is best for them. Should they try to start running again, even though they really don't enjoy it? Should they drag themselves to the community pool for laps in the morning, even though getting up that early is painful? Maybe they should hire a trainer they can't afford. Uh, no. This does not have to be hard, and it surely does not have to be painful! Exercise (a.k.a. movement) should not be something you dread. Even if you think you are the kind of person who "hates" exercise, you at least have to move to exist as a human on this earth. There is undoubtedly *something* out there that we can find for you to do that you enjoy and that will get you moving.

If you really are starting from square one with the whole idea of movement on a regular basis, take some time to do some discovery work on what might be a good fit. Maybe start by thinking about what you enjoyed as a kid. If you didn't play sports and spent most of your time inside, why? Did you feel intimidated by other kids? Did you just prefer to have your head in a book? Either way, was there something, anything, you enjoyed doing? Riding your bike to school? Going swimming in the summer? Anything? Start with just one movement that wasn't awful, and go from there.

When I was a preteen, my dad got my brother and me tennis racquets and lessons. I vaguely remembered liking it but not loving it. For those of you who haven't been on a tennis court, it is generally about 15 degrees warmer on it than around it. So a typical 100° day in El Paso, Texas, puts the courts at about 115°. Let's just say my whiny preteen self was not really "feeling it." But last year, I was just so tired of working out at home due to the pandemic and really wanted to do some socially distanced but friendly activity that I could get into. I found a lovely instructor who works at a community court just a few blocks from my house, got myself a basic racquet, and off to the races I went. I loved learning something new! I really loved how I had to be fully mentally engaged in every movement lest I get reprimanded for my lack of effort. Now that I've been doing it for about a year, I find that I'm really enjoying learning the strategy of the game and the power I didn't know my old rotator cuff had. My point is, I decided to try something completely different from what I'd been doing my whole adult life and found a sport that I truly love! Added plus: I get a killer workout without even thinking about it.

Keep It Fresh

I actually encourage you to find a handful of things you like doing. Our bodies are incredibly smart and quickly adapt to become more efficient at the activities we do. By varying your movement practices, you will find a myriad of benefits: quicker fitness gains, fewer injuries, and of course, a lower chance of getting bored out of your mind! I realize that for some of you, it might be hard to find even one thing that you find interesting to do movement-wise. But once you do, I think you'll find it becomes easier to come up with another and another. For example, if you like swimming, maybe try a water aerobics/fitness class. If you like going for long walks, maybe try your hand at swinging a golf club. If you love golfing, maybe pick up a tennis racquet. You get the idea. Just keep your mind open to the possibility you might like a few different things, and then try them all. There's no harm in giving it a shot once and just seeing how you feel about it. You can always ditch it and never do it again. But you might just stumble on something that you really love.

When you move your body in different ways from day to day or season to season, you'll find that you achieve a

When you move your body in different ways from day to day or season to season, you'll find that you achieve a level of fitness you never thought possible.

level of fitness you never thought possible. Why? Because humans need a variety of movements just like we need a variety of vegetables in our diet. We need to go forward, backward, sideways, rotate, bend, and reach. We need to go fast, slow, and even stop. If you are moving in the same direction every time you exercise, at a similar cadence, on the same terrain, you likely will top out your fitness potential very quickly—not to mention increase your chances of injury. But if on Monday and Friday, you run hills, Tuesday and Saturday you swim, Wednesday you do yoga, and Sunday keep your standing play-date with your grandkids, you will be one fit grandparent!

Where I see a lot of people get in trouble is they find that one thing they love doing and never do anything else. At the beginning, they see amazing changes in their bodies. Maybe they lose weight; maybe they feel their muscles in ways they never have before. But after several weeks, that progress stagnates, and they find homeostasis.

Their bodies have become more efficient at the movement, and now it takes less effort (less caloric burn) to do the exact same activity as when they started. Our bodies are designed to preserve energy. We may have access to all we will ever need, but our ancient-built physiques don't know that. All they know is that suddenly they had to learn to do something hard that required a high expenditure of energy, and it was hard to recover from. Our bodies quickly figure out what muscles to use and in what way so as to make that activity as energy-cheap as possible. As I said, the human body is wicked smart!

Years ago, my husband was fed up with being overweight and slowly started a running routine. He was working out with me using weights and doing a variety of things at the gym but added the running in for cardiovascular work. We live close to Stanford University, which has a great trail referred to as "The Dish" where a giant satellite sits at the top of a hill overlooking the Bay Area. It is 3.7 miles of glorious hills. He would run that thing in circles over and over again. The repetition of the same loop, with all the ups and downs within, was perfect for helping him get into almost a meditative state while pounding that trail. A couple of times, he even looped it seven times to get a marathon. He was in the shape of his life!

That was ten years ago, and while he still ran it quite a bit—one hundred miles a month on that same loop, the variety in his workouts began to wane. Work got very busy for him as the pandemic hit, and he was sometimes putting in sixteen-hour days. But he still ran. And yet his weight crept up a good twenty pounds. He still ran. Slowly, minor injuries started to set in: sore Achilles' and tight back. It had stopped working for him. His amazing runner's body was so efficient at cruising around that loop that he no longer burned much energy to make it happen. It was time for variety. Since then, he has cut *way* back on running—a measly two to six miles a week, mostly in sprints on a treadmill. He has added boot camps, personal training, and workouts with friends. The weight is coming off, and the aches and pains are going away. Variety was exactly what his body needed!

I use him as an example because of how extreme it was. But you don't have to be doing one hundred miles a month on the same loop to lose effectiveness in your workouts and stop seeing results. Just walking your dog around the same loop in your neighborhood every day is going to lose its luster. Your dog will get bored too. ***You can have a favorite thing you do. Just don't do it every day, and try not to do it in exactly the same way.***

My husband is also a good example of the addictiveness of exercise. A few of you may roll your eyes at the idea that exercise can be addictive. In fact, you may say that you hate exercise. You may be right. But once you feel how a certain movement leaves you feeling almost high—feeling like all your problems are suddenly smaller, like you just got a shot of the best drugs ever—you'll be hooked. I know people who feel this way about their morning walk, their yoga practice, and the laps they do in their home pool. They just have to do it. I have felt this way about running (not so much these days), about lifting weights at the gym, about yoga, and now about my tennis lessons. You'll know you have finally tripped on a movement practice that is right for you when you finally get that "high." When you walk away from that workout and go, "Wow, that was fun!" And even more so when you feel compelled to do it again and again.

> You can have a favorite thing you do. Just don't do it every day, and try not to do it in exactly the same way.

When you find that "one" thing, get excited! That's the one activity you can always go to. When you aren't in the mood to do exercise for the sake of exercise. For some, this will be something that pulls you out of your head and into the moment. Especially when an activity is new to you, it will require that you really focus on how you're moving your body. You might need to focus on whether your breathing is right or how your posture is. You may have to be focused on injuries that you're nursing or preventing. When I'm taking a tennis lesson, I can't think about what I'm making for dinner or how we are going to find the money for the mortgage payment. I have to think about how I'm holding the racquet, what type of swing I'm about to make, how much power to generate, and where I want the ball to land.

Other activities may become addictive in that they allow you the brain space to really think about your life. When I used to run a lot, I used that time for all kinds of meditations: noodling on a dilemma in my life, planning out the next steps in a work project, and considering how I could have handled an issue better after the fact. Other times I would just have really great music on and focus on how to get my feet to match the beat of the track. Occasionally, you might find me belting out a few tunes or doing an epic drum solo as I made my way down the street.

Whatever the reason, I hope that you find something(s) that compels you to keep going. To need to do it again and again. To put in just five more minutes. And if you start getting in better shape at the same time, that's a great added bonus. You'll notice I haven't spoken much yet about the fitness aspect of movement. Instead, I find it most important to focus on the emotional, social, and even spiritual aspects. *If you feel better as a human in your skin because of the movement practices you engage in, you are far more likely to stick with them over the long term.* You'll be more willing to keep up your weekend walks with a friend, or group yoga class, or solo run because it's "who you are and what you do" than if you just like the way it makes you look.

I've been teaching fitness for decades now. I have taught all manner of boot camps, yoga, pilates, and personal training. The people who came to those sessions time and time again were not in the best shape. They didn't look like fitness models. They didn't have washboard abs. They were people who liked the movements we were doing and the way they felt when they finished. These devotees knew that no matter what mood they were in when they came in, they'd leave feeling better. This is such an integral part of what I do that I use it as a benchmark every time I teach. When I see someone walk in with slumped shoulders and a foggy disposition, I make it my mission to get them breathing right and engage their mind in the activity. And when I see them walk out the door standing taller and smiling, it is the best type of success. *Knowing that just moving, engaging, and breathing can completely alter the trajectory of one person's day is why exercise is addictive.* That is why

If you feel better as a human in your skin because of the movement practices you engage in, you are far more likely to stick with them over the long term.

137

Knowing that just moving, engaging, and breathing can complely alter the trajectory of one person's day is why exercise is addictive.

I show up every day to do this again and again. My "why" to move can also be your "why."

The First Mile

Getting started (with most anything) is the hardest part. Whether you're trying a new diet program or getting ready to train for a marathon, getting started is the absolute biggest hurdle. When prospective clients reach out to me to inquire about my services and next steps, I make sure to remind them that they've already done the hardest part: realizing they need help and seeking it. Once we get that first appointment going, we can build momentum. But breaking that inertia—that's the hard part.

My husband often jokes with our children, ***"Do something! Even if it's wrong!"*** Meaning: Get off your bum and go! Sitting around and hoping for things to be different is not going to get it. Sometimes it doesn't even matter if it's the wrong choice. Who cares if the first activity you pick ends up being awful and you never do it again? You've already broken the inertia. You can now more easily course correct and find a better option. It will be less daunting than the first time you had to rip the Band-Aid off and get going.

"Do something! Even if it's wrong!"

Once you find something you like (or even that you don't detest), getting started will still be the hardest part. Every time. When I'm in the habit of running, that first mile is always a doozy. I often have to mentally coach myself to just get my shoes on and get in one mile. Just one. I promise myself that if I finish that one mile, I can stop and walk. At least 90 percent of the time, I feel pretty good after that first mile and choose to keep going a bit. This goes for all my movement activities: just getting on the bike, just carving out the time to get on my

You just have to start.

yoga mat, just signing up for that boot camp. Once I set the wheels in motion, it goes just fine. *You just have to start.*

Use Your "Why"

Go back to the beginning of this section, where we had you revisit your goals and "why." If you are having a hard time with those first steps, remembering why you are doing it (whatever it is) is critical. If you need to get moving to prevent heart disease and not leave your family missing you, that should be a pretty compelling reminder of why you might want to lace up those sneakers. If you have found yourself bailing time and again on your activities because it was inconvenient or you just keep procrastinating, you have to remember *why!* In fact, you might want to take your most important "why" and write it in big block letters and post it somewhere you will be reminded. Maybe you need it in your closet right above your running shoes, or on top of your dresser where you keep that swimsuit. You know where it needs to go.

Don't feel bad or beat yourself up for being challenged with getting started. Trust me, you are not alone! I know hardcore athletes who still struggle with keeping up their training routines or starting new diets. ***Human nature is self-preservation.*** Just like our ancestors didn't have to "exercise" to burn calories, neither did they burn energy, if not requisite. Those genes haven't changed. Our bodies still assume that if we have all the things we need to live comfortably, there is no reason to work harder. The problem is that we are missing such a critical element of health if we don't now force ourselves to move on a regular basis.

> # Human nature is self-preservation.

Key Elements of Your Movement Practice

So we've faced the challenge of why you need to move. You are bracing for the *getting started* bit. But what in the heck will you choose to do? First of all, let's not make this hard. One of the many reasons people hire a personal trainer is they want someone to fine-tune their program without having to spend too much time thinking about it themselves. But what personal trainers do when it comes to program design is not magic. Yes, many of us have spent years in school learning the precise combination of movements to help clients achieve their goals. But in all honesty, it can be boiled down to five simple categories that most all humans should incorporate:

Get Your Heart Rate Up
Get and Stay Strong
Keep Your Balance
Don't Get Too Tight
Rest and Recover

It's really that simple. Let me break these down for you a bit. Then I'll help you figure out how much of each category and when to incorporate them into your routines.

Get your heart rate up.

Or, as some people refer to it: "cardio." I really don't like that term. I mean, if your heart isn't pumping, you're done. So yes, we can get the heart stronger, but there are so many ways to do that. For our purposes here, let's stick with the simplicity of just "get your heart rate up." If left to our own devices, most of us wouldn't feel our hearts pounding unless we were in imminent danger, or the elevator was broken on the way to the 20th floor. *Humans are designed to do two things: move for long distances at a moderate/slow pace and occasionally run like crazy.* That's pretty much it! So when it comes to incorporating "cardio" into your workout routine, you need to keep those two things in mind.

> # Humans are designed to do two things: move for long distances at a moderate/slow pace and occasionally run like crazy.

Again, go back to the movements you enjoy. If you are a swimmer, for example, maybe you swim laps at a moderate pace once or twice a week for an hour. Then once a week, you swim for only twenty minutes but spend ten of them alternating between the fastest you can crawl one lap and a slow recovery the next. If you just like walking, the same thing. You walk at a moderate pace on your favorite scenic route for your longer walks two to three times per week, then once a week you tackle some speed intervals. To do this, just find something to look at in the distance (a tree, a parked car, etc.), get to it as quickly as your legs will allow, then go back to a normal pace until you are breathing normally. These shorter, more intense bouts should only last for a total of only twenty to thirty minutes. This includes warming up.

What I just described is the basic idea behind interval training. Some of you may have heard the term "high intensity interval training" or HIIT. This is a fabulous way to train your heart to pump out serious amounts of blood to your extremities for a few seconds (15–45) and then (and most importantly) recover! If you incorporate intervals like these into your workouts twice per week, you will be stunned at your increase in energy. This action of training the cardiovascular system to kick into high gear and then back to low not only gets your heart stronger but also increases metabolism.[9] You'll find that one twenty-minute session will leave you beaming for hours afterward. The only caveat is that you don't want to do it every day. ***The whole point is to give those short intervals your all and then recover.*** When you let your system recover, it grows stronger! So on alternate days, you do some low and slow movements like scenic cycling or walks with friends.

> The whole point is to give those short intervals your *all* and then recover.

For most of your cardiovascular activities, you just want to focus on your basic hikes, bike rides, and so on. Then about two days a week, you'll incorporate a few minutes of intervals. Again, make sure that you don't do super long intervals, or you won't get the results you want. Keep those intense outputs to less than sixty seconds but actually closer to thirty.[10] There's a fine line between putting positive stress on your heart and putting additional excessive stress on it. Also, if you think you are too old or too deconditioned to do intervals, you are wrong! I have clients who do intervals just by sitting in a chair and pumping their arms up and down. You can do it on a recumbent bike, on a treadmill, or anywhere. You just have to find a movement, any movement, that you can do that will get your heart rate up for a few seconds. Then stop, or go slow until you feel recovered, then do it again. Repeat eight to ten times and you're done. It's that easy.

Get and stay strong.

Again, we can make the program design very intricate and confusing, or we can keep it simple. Whether you are a six-foot male wanting to pack on pounds of muscle or a ninety-year-old woman trying to keep her bones from breaking, you all need to be strong, relative to your life and goals. This might mean deadlifting three hundred pounds or picking up a bottle of water over your head a few times. Regardless of where you are starting and where you are trying to go, you'll need to incorporate these four basic movements into your routine:

- Push
- Rotate
- Isometrics
- Pull

When I was a brand-new trainer, I used to sit up at night plotting out every step of every workout I would be giving the next day. Invariably, that client would show up and tell me about a new injury or tell me they were underslept and not in the mood to be pushed, or whatever. I would have to scrap my plans and play it by ear. After a while, I realized that all I had to do was keep these four basics in mind as I built a circuit for them, and off we went. By incorporating a push, rotation, isometrics, and a pull into a routine, you will likely get your targeted muscle groups from all angles. You'll get a full range of motion and core engagement. Your muscles will also be used in all the ways Mother Nature intended. The only hard part is figuring out which exercises to plug in.

I will walk you through the process below. However, as a thank-you for picking up this book, I have put a secret page on my website for you. There you will find several videos showing you a few workout routines. There is one for general toning, one for beginners, and one for showing you how to really advance your workouts. You can access these and more at dfitlife.com/own-your-wellness-resources.

Pushing:

This is as simple as it sounds. Anything that requires you to move things away from you is a push. Pushups, yes, but also things like overhead presses, chest presses, leg presses, squats, chest flies and tricep presses. In general, all pushing movements will engage muscles like your triceps, chest, shoulders, quadriceps, and, of course, your core. *I put pushing movements at the top of the list because they usually incorporate muscles that we already use all day.* If you are stuck on the computer, driving, and so on, you are already overusing these muscles and movements. While it will be important for you to build strength and range of motion, we don't want to end your workout with more pushes. I think it's best for us to finish a workout with moves that leave us open, upright, and breathing well. Here are examples of two simple pushing movements: an elevated push-up and a squat-to-overhead press.

> I put pushing movements at the top of the list because they usually incorporate muscles that we already use all day.

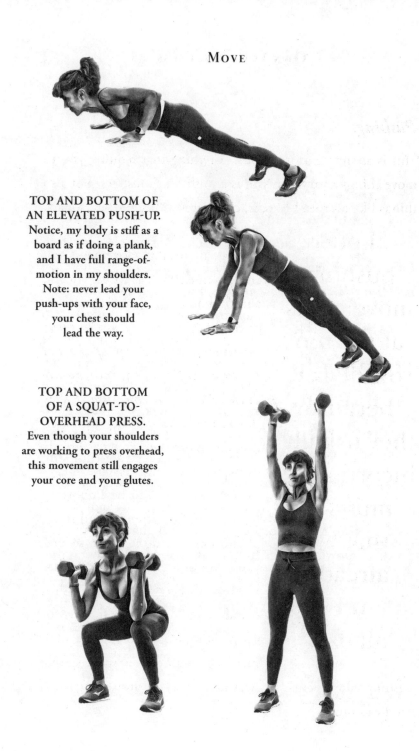

TOP AND BOTTOM OF AN ELEVATED PUSH-UP. Notice, my body is stiff as a board as if doing a plank, and I have full range-of-motion in my shoulders. Note: never lead your push-ups with your face, your chest should lead the way.

TOP AND BOTTOM OF A SQUAT-TO-OVERHEAD PRESS. Even though your shoulders are working to press overhead, this movement still engages your core and your glutes.

Rotating:

This is one of those things that we just lose if we don't use it. It is also one of the movements that a lot of people don't even think about when it comes to working out. And why not? *We need rotation for almost all movements:* hip and ankle rotation to walk and run; thoracic (rib cage area) and shoulder rotation for throwing, reaching, and pulling; and cervical (neck) rotation to look over your shoulder. Without a good range of motion and/or rotation in all these areas, we end up stiff, weak, and out of balance. Exercises that target rotation often are good stretches too. I like to do big sweeping movements with my arms in all directions, lunge in all different ways, and practice throwing things from both sides of my body.

> We need rotation for almost all movements

**START AND END OF A
LOWER-BODY CORE TWIST.**
Shoulders should stay flush
with the floor, hips and
knees at 90º.

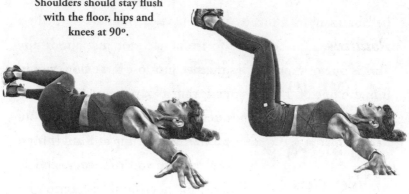

**BOTTOM AND TOP OF A
WEIGHTED SQUAT WITH
A DIAGONAL CHOP.**
Rotation should be coming from
the ground up: ankles, hips, and
shoulders working together.

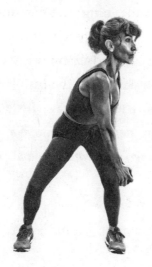
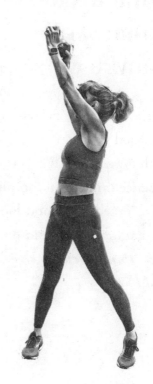

149

Isometrics:

This just means holding your muscles while contracted and not moving. For example, you might hold a dumbbell halfway in a biceps curl. Or you could stay still in a plank position. You can do isometrics for just about any muscle group, but *why* would you want to do these? First of all, one of the most common uses of human strength is to hold things: children, groceries, boxes, and so on. You need both strength and endurance to hold things for long periods of time. In addition, the "core" muscles are designed to be like little Energizer bunnies and just keep going, and going, and going, and going ... We don't want our tummy, back, and bum muscles giving out on us when we are trying to accomplish hard things. It is possible to have toned and good-looking muscles that have little or no endurance to hold on for long periods of time. *So, in addition to getting strong, we need to make sure we can hold on!*

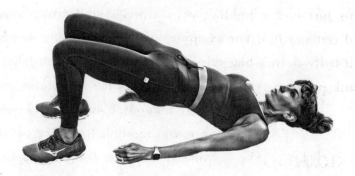

BRIDGE POSITION. The toes and knees should be pointing straight ahead. Muscles engaged should include the hamstrings, glutes, back, and even the back of the shoulders.

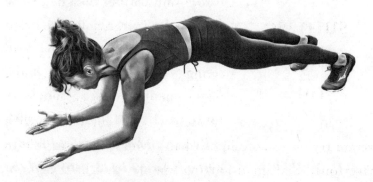

PLANK POSITION. In my preferred variation, the palms are turned up to keep the shoulders open, the head is aligned with the spine (not tilted up or down), the glutes are engaged, and the belly button is drawn in. This can be done from your knees as well.

Pulling:

I like to save the best for last, and workouts are no exception. Pulling movements are unfortunately lacking in our modern society. We spend all day forward on our computers and phones. Then we maybe go for a walk or bike ride and aim forward the whole time. Maybe we will sit on the couch and watch TV, and our heads are jutting forward again. We need to get the whole back end working far more than it does, and all we have to do is pull on things. Pulling movements like rows, deadlifts, and curls target the muscles in your shoulders, back, rear end, and hamstrings. I love seeing people leave their workouts standing taller, shoulders rolled back, and head high. *We get that alpha, the world-is-my-oyster, posture by targeting all the muscles on the back side of your gorgeous body!*

> We get that alpha, the world-is-my-oyster, posture by targeting all the muscles on the back side of your gorgeous body!

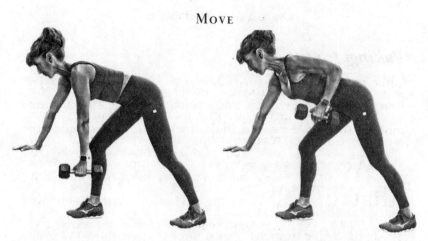

START AND END OF A SUPPORTED DUMBBELL ROW. Notice, I'm supported at a level that allows me to keep my back flat and core engaged. The movement should initiate from your shoulder blades, and the elbow should come up just past your waist.

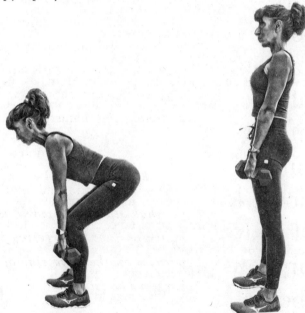

BOTTOM AND TOP OF A DUMBBELL DEAD LIFT. What's most important here are the flat back and hinge of my hips. The dumbbell should stay close to the body as you slide from start to finish. The head should stay in alignment with the spine.

153

Putting It All Together

Now all you have to do is take an exercise from each of the above categories and put them into a plan for the week. For my clients who have time to do strength training only twice a week, I like to do an exercise of each category in a circuit, meaning you do one push, one rotation, one isometric, and one pull exercise. Then you repeat those in the same order two to three times through. If you have time to strength train three or more times per week (I do not recommend more than four), you might break them down into groups. For example, Mondays are push and pull; Wednesdays are rotation and isometrics, and Saturdays are only pulling again. Just an idea, but you get the gist. The key is that you put in about forty-eight hours to recover between hitting the same movement and muscle groups again. So maybe you put your low and slow heart rate day in between doing two days of strength training.

You can also vary the intensity and duration of your strength sets. For someone who wants to just be somewhat toned and reasonably strong, I'd recommend anywhere from ten to fifteen repetitions at a resistance that seems doable but challenging. For this person, maybe doing a bodyweight squat is plenty challenging for fifteen repetitions. But lifting only two pounds overhead is too easy. If you could do thirty repetitions, you should make it harder. If you can do only five, it's too much and increases your risk of injury. Just aim for weight or intensity that allows you to stay in that ten to twenty range. For someone who is advanced in their lifting techniques and wants to work on strength, they would want to move weights around that challenge them at a mere five to ten reps. Don't do more, and if you can't do two, you really need to throttle back. Note, for isometric exercises, you will work on how long you can hold the contraction with good form. Here are some repetition and set ranges you can aim for based on your goals:

- Strength: 5–10 reps for 2–4 sets
- Toning: 10–15 for 3–5 sets
- Endurance: 15–25 reps for 1–3 sets

Note: These are ranges I have developed anecdotally over the years from my own workouts, and those of hundreds of clients.

Before embarking on your weight training, make sure you've "warmed up" from the day: maybe you've taken the dog for a walk, done some housework already, and so on. Start with a trial set of each exercise you've chosen with either no weights at all, or very light weights. You want to take your joints and body through the full range of motion you are getting ready for. Then start your sets. Again, depending on your goal, you'll do one exercise, then go to the next. Once you do them all, maybe you have time to repeat another set (round) or two. You can increase the toughness if you feel like the first set was too easy. You can also back off if it was overkill. Use the repetition and set ranges above to guide you. You want to do enough to elicit

I promise: if you give yourself a day or two of letting those muscles recover, they will grow and develop faster than you could ever imagine!

a repair response (and growth) from your muscle fibers but not so much as to injure yourself. Then *rest!* Please. Have a good meal. Drink some water. *I promise: if you give yourself a day or two of letting those muscles recover, they will grow and develop faster than you could ever imagine!*

Again, keep it simple, listen to your body, and respect what it tells you. If at any point you feel pain, *stop*. Your body is smart. It knows when something is wrong. Please do not disregard its wisdom. And that rest I keep insisting on, it will help you heal and repair. You will have fewer injuries and many years of getting strong to look forward to.

Keep your balance.

I mean, shouldn't this be a goal for all of us? Really, the alternative to having balance is generally falling over, and that is not what we are going for. Many people think that balance is just something we are bound to lose as we get older. Wrong. We are

bound to lose the use of pretty much any skill we don't practice. I grew up a fluent Spanish speaker living on the border in
El Paso, Texas. But when I moved away at age eleven and didn't
speak a word of it for years, I lost almost all I had once known.
**Any skill, including balancing, requires regular and progres-
sive practice.**

One of the first things I ask clients to do when it comes to improving balance is to take their shoes off. I know, it sounds crazy, but you have tons of tiny little muscles and nerves in your feet that really need to *feel* the ground. When we bind our feet up in cushy sneakers and thick socks, we turn off the foot's natural ability to use the

Any skill, including balancing, requires regular and progressive practice.

ground to react to. So start barefoot first thing in the morning.
My favorite time and place to get people started with regular
balance practice is while brushing their teeth. Stand barefoot
at your sink, spread your toes as wide as you can (yes, this is a
good skill, and the spread helps you hold onto the floor), and
stand tall. Maybe you start there on two feet. But if you are
ready for a challenge, lift a foot up while you brush your top
teeth. Squeeze your bum on that standing leg, and keep your
posture tall. When you switch to the bottom teeth, switch your
feet. If you do this every time you brush your teeth, you have a
built-in twice-a-day practice.

Once things like standing on one leg are easy for you, you can progress to movement on one leg. You can try reaching for something on the counter in front of you. You can try moving your head (and your gaze) side to side or up and down. Think of things you do on a daily basis that require extra balance effort: walking up or down stairs, hiking on uneven terrain, and so on. Then you can try to replicate those movements when you're exercising too. Maybe you take one of your pull/rotate/isolate/push exercises and try it on one leg or on your toes. Heck, maybe just try closing your eyes. That one gets me every time.

One of the main reasons you see elderly people shuffle is not because they have just lost strength but because they've lost balance. In order to walk without shuffling, you have to be able to briefly pick one foot up off the ground as the other takes that next step. When this skill is lost, you end up trying to walk while keeping both feet on the ground. So start practicing *now*. And if you find that you are already shuffling, start practicing balance. ***You can regain it.*** Just start easy and safely, and work your way up. Start by standing against a counter on two feet, and close your eyes. Hold on to the counter, or keep it close so you don't fall. How long can you go without feeling like you need to open your eyes? Once that's easy, try it with your eyes open, and just pick up the heel of one foot (using the toes like a kickstand). Once you

You can regain it.

can hold the balance on each foot like that, try lifting the whole foot up. You get the idea. I have seen clients regain balance to a level they would never have thought possible, and you can too!

For those of you who are balance pros, you too can add difficulty by doing single-legged exercises with your eyes shut. You can also try standing on uneven surfaces to challenge yourself even further. There is no need to go nuts with all the balls and beams and whatnot. If I see one more stupid video of a trainer having a client stand on a giant physioball while lifting a heavy weight, I'm going to scream. Nowhere in normal life is that required unless you are trying out for a role in Cirque du Soleil. You'll only be setting yourself up for injury, and that is never the goal. *As I said earlier, think about things that happen in your life that are challenging balance-wise, and try to replicate those in your workouts.*

Think about things that happen in your life that are challenging balance-wise, and try to replicate those in your workouts.

Don't get too tight.

Yeah, that's really the whole goal of stretching. It's not to be Gumby (sorry to you young'uns who don't recognize that reference). In fact, being too flexible (aka, hypermobile) is a real issue for many people. If you are one of those (and you know who you are), your main goal is to get strong and stay strong to prevent those joints from being too lax. For the rest of us, the real focus is just on not getting too tight.

First of all, you have to understand that we get tightness in our bodies for generally one of two reasons: (1) Our joints don't get nutrients and hydration unless they move. That's why we are stiff in the morning and why people who have arthritis often feel better once they get moving. By using the muscles and tendons that pull across the joint in question, blood flow increases to the area, and the necessary nutrients are brought to that joint. (2) Our innately brilliant bodies know when to protect themselves. If you notice new or unusual tightness in an area, it's likely because your body is trying to prevent further injury in that spot. For example, you wake up with a serious crick in your neck. You likely had your head in a horrific position for way too long while sleeping, and now all the muscles that surround that area are stiff and tight. Your body clamped that area down so that it can heal. This is not a time to force yourself into a neck stretch. You know that being ginger with it and maybe applying some heat will help you get back to normal soon.

Regardless of why you are tight, you'll want to focus your energy on stretching areas that can really make a difference in your overall wellness. To do this, you want to think about how all your body parts are connected. Yes, we have muscles and tendons that cross over every joint, but we also have connective tissue called fascia that weaves all over our body in different fascial lines. These fascial lines are like interstate highways that connect your head to your feet, or your shoulder to your hip. You have a fascial line that weaves from your eyebrows, over your head, and down to the soles of your feet. This posterior fascial line connects everything on your back end and is why when you have tight hamstrings, you might also have a tight back (and vice versa). There are fascial lines that run diagonally from one shoulder across the opposite hip. You can see some examples of fascial lines below:

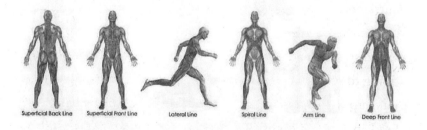

Superficial Back Line   Superficial Front Line   Lateral Line   Spiral Line   Arm Line   Deep Front Line

http://simplybowentherapy.com.au/wp-content/uploads
/2017/04/fascia-lines.png

Once you figure out where your tightness is centered, you'll want to do stretches that incorporate the fascial lines that joint or joints are in. Here's a good example: you might be tight in your right hamstring (back of your thigh). So you would want to stretch from under your left foot, up the back of your leg, all the way up to your opposite shoulder. In fact, the positions I'm in below are my favorite ways to stretch hamstrings as they loosen up the fascial lines all along the posterior diagonal.

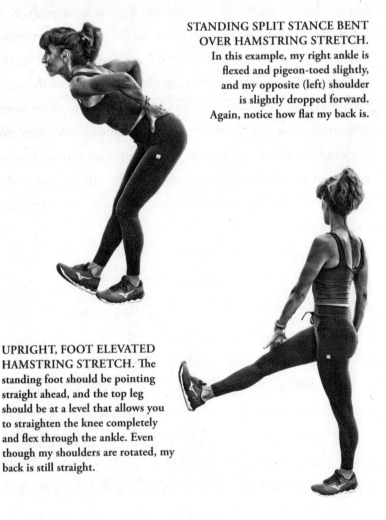

STANDING SPLIT STANCE BENT OVER HAMSTRING STRETCH. In this example, my right ankle is flexed and pigeon-toed slightly, and my opposite (left) shoulder is slightly dropped forward. Again, notice how flat my back is.

UPRIGHT, FOOT ELEVATED HAMSTRING STRETCH. The standing foot should be pointing straight ahead, and the top leg should be at a level that allows you to straighten the knee completely and flex through the ankle. Even though my shoulders are rotated, my back is still straight.

This concept can be a little confusing. So once again, as a thank you for picking this up, see additional stretch examples at dfitlife.com/own-your-wellness-resources.

Of course, there are many ways to stretch. You can do yoga, you can take classes, you can use a foam roller or a massage ball. What matters is that you don't add insult to injury. Find a modality that suits you and stick with it. I am a super-bendy person (in most directions), so stretching doesn't really work that well for me, even when I feel tight. For me, using a foam roller or a lacrosse ball against the wall is much more effective. I can target tight areas with pressure and then work the muscles around it into a full range of motion. Regardless of the type of stretching your body needs, make sure not to engage in intense stretches when your body is cold. Like I said, joints don't get lubricated until you get them moving. So go for a walk, do some Tai Chi, or get some housework done before you start your stretches.

Rest and recover.

Please do not skip this part. Rest and recovery are a sorely underappreciated piece of the health puzzle. I swear this is the absolute hardest part of each and every one of my client's movement practices. Getting people to let go of the idea that more is better is counterintuitive. I have struggled with it myself over the years and continue to. I constantly have to remind myself that doing more Peloton classes or

I know, I know, this doesn't sound right, but let me tell you, sometimes doing less is exactly what the doctor ordered.

more core workouts not only doesn't help me look lean and toned but it can actually make me gain weight and stay soft. *I know, I know, this doesn't sound right, but let me tell you, sometimes doing less is exactly what the doctor ordered.*

I have two types of clients that fall prey to the "more is more" mentality and do themselves a disservice: men, like all of them (sorry, but it's true), and women in their perimenopausal and menopausal years. While both groups of people are struggling with different health challenges and health goals, they seem to suffer from the same mentality: "I guess what I did when I was younger isn't enough anymore; I need to do more." Sadly, they pack on more pounds and lose, not gain, muscle tone. But why? Why does this strategy backfire every time?

Well, that's because the magic is in the rest. When your muscles, joints, cardiovascular system, and even brain get to fully recover, they come back stronger. Conversely, when you pound the pavement daily, do the same weight routine, or sacrifice sleep for another morning run, you just break yourself down. Chronic exercisers often end up with nagging injuries, blood sugar dysregulation, sleep disturbances, and a whole host of issues related to the long-term stress that over-training causes. In fact, when you neglect rest and recovery, your workouts go from being a hormetic (good) stressor to becoming yet another strain on your body, mind, and poor overworked adrenal glands.

So, what is the right balance of rest and work? This actually doesn't have to be complicated. The basic idea is that if you move one way one day, that movement and the muscles involved with it need a day off, sometimes two. It's literally that simple. You know that feeling of muscle soreness the day after a good workout? That is the result of breaking down the muscle tissue. When you nourish your-self with sufficient protein to rebuild those muscles, you see them tone up and even grow. However, if you go back to working out the same muscles the next day and break them down again, you never get time to recover. If you've ever heard the term "catabolic," this is what it's referring to. You are putting your body into a state of breaking down, not building up.

Instead, you want to aim for being "anabolic." There's a reason you just thought of steroids and bodybuilders when you read that word. Anabolic means you are building up and growing. Back in my fleeting stint in figure competi-tion, it was drilled into me to put at least forty-eight hours between training the same muscle groups. I would train one area, say my back muscles, to complete fatigue and intense ensuing soreness. Then, the next day, I would train my chest muscles. Then, core and legs. And then rotate through them all throughout the week. That way, I was always allowing those micro tears in the muscle to repair and grow. The result was about seventeen pounds of solid muscle in just a few months. In fact, you can think of recovery as Miracle-Gro for your body.

Now, you might be thinking that this doesn't apply to you since putting on muscle isn't one of your goals. But if you're trying to avoid injury, increase your energy, build your stamina, or really improve your health in any way, rest and recovery are still critical to your movement practice. Even if you are just walking long trails every day, you need to find a way to vary your movements from day to day so that you're not just moving in that same sagittal (straight ahead) plane all the time. Maybe work in a swim or yoga a few times per week. Regardless of your goals, please work in time to recover.

The Key Elements of Your Movement

The "key elements of your movement" all work together to help you "own your wellness." They are all interconnected. Below, I have made a chart that helps you line up all the elements, why, how, and when to do them.

	Why	Format	Frequency
Get Your Heart Rate Up	*Condition the heart for both long-duration activities and short bouts of intense output.*	*Low and slow: any enjoyable activity with a consistent moderate output.* *Intervals: 5 minute warm-up, 10–15 minutes of alternating highest output for 15–45 seconds with active recovery until heart rate normalizes.*	*Low and slow: 3–4 days per week for 30–90 minutes.* *Intervals: Start with once per week and increase to 2–3 times per week with no less than 48 hours between sessions.*
Get and Stay Strong	*Maintain posture, increase muscle tone, increase bone density, etc.*	*Push, rotate, isolate, and pull.* *5–10, 10–15, or 15–20 reps per exercise.* *2–5 sets.* *About 30 minutes*	*2–4 times per week*
Keep Your Balance	*To be fully functional your whole life and not fall down!*	*Start easy, and try being barefoot.* *Add challenge with eyes closed, moving your head, and changing the stimulus under your feet.*	*As often as you can. We need balance all day, so you can and should practice whenever possible.* *Remember the teeth-brushing ;)*
Don't Get Too Tight	*To prevent injury and keep a good range of motion.*	*After a warm-up, target tight areas along fascial lines.* *You can hold stretches, use foam rollers or balls, and even do a yoga class.*	*After most workouts or any time your body feels stiff.*
Rest and Recover	*To allow your muscles, joints, and cardiovascular system to gain strength and improve.*	*Either taking time off completely or doing complementary movements on alternate days.*	*Ideally 24–48 hours' rest for each muscle group or movement.*

Train in the Posture You Aspire To

I'd like to interject a little note here about form. One of the main reasons people seek out a personal trainer is to watch their "form." When I think of someone's "form" in the context of exercise, I'm thinking about how this movement *should* look. How *should* this person function? People don't come to me to end up with even more hunched shoulders or caved-in rear ends. They come to me to look strong, upright, balanced, and confident. So if you want to stand tall and function in a pain-free body all day, then you should make sure all your movements are done in that aspirational form. If you'd prefer to look like a roly-poly or a turtle, then by all means, please stay slumped on the couch looking at your laptop. Get my drift?

In general, proper posture in all movement would include attention to the following:

- Alignment: Head over shoulders; shoulders over hips; hips over ankles

- Engagement: Really thinking about the muscles you are using and how they are working

- Support: Having a good core engagement to support the movement you are doing (more on this below).

And don't be afraid to use a mirror! There's a reason they are all over the gym. Aside from vanity, mirrors can be very helpful in figuring out how to position yourself. Some of my clients just hate using a mirror and rely on me watching their form, which is fine. But regardless of how you feel about what you see in the mirror, I encourage you to use it as a tool to ensure your form is spot on.

Your Core

The term "core" is both overused and misunderstood. It seems like every new fitness studio has the word "core" in its name. Every group class is some variation of "core work." So we all end up thinking we are focusing on core, but do we really know what that even means? I'll tell you what it's not: your abs. Yes, your ab muscles are part of your core, but those sexy six-pack abs have very little to do with having a strong and supportive trunk for optimal human function. *Your core includes everything from your shoulders to your hips: front-to-back, side-to-side, and all around.* Remember those fascial lines we learned about earlier? They all run part-way through your core. We need a strong "core" because without one, our arms and legs would be pretty much floundering.

> Your core includes everything from your shouldners to your hips: front to back, side to side, and all around.

One of the easiest examples I have for you of why we need a strong core is rotator cuff injuries. Likely you, or someone you know, have dealt with pain or injury in the "rotator cuff."

While these injuries are quite common, they often are the result of a weak core and incorrect posture. When you reach out and don't have your shoulder anchored into your rib cage, engaging all the core muscles surrounding that area, you don't have a good base of support for that reach. Imagine a diving board. The really tall and long ones protrude from a very solid base anchored into the concrete surrounding the pool. Now imagine taking just the board and laying one end on the floor next to the pool and letting the other half jut over the water. If you dared to walk down that plank toward the water, it would just collapse. The muscles you have around your rib cage act like the solid base of a diving board. When you reach out to lift something far away from your body, anchoring into your core lends amazing strength to the limb doing the work.

How should you train your core?

Well, not the way most of us think. I would venture to guess that most of us picture lying on a ball and doing crunches or holding our head while we bicycle our legs. When exactly on a normal day would any human need to do things like that? Never! Your core is designed to work for long periods of time, sustaining a base for your limbs to work off of. The core muscles need not only strength but endurance. Most of us can correct our sitting or standing posture for a moment, but how long can we sustain that? Sadly, for many, not long. *Ideally, a strong core would allow you to sit upright without fatigue, walk tall for miles on end, and engage in sports with power to your limbs in all directions.*

When we discussed strength training before, one of the "four basic movements" was isometric holds. Your core muscles *really* need isometric work. Since your core muscles need to be able to stay strong for long periods of time, we would want to train those muscles to withstand resistance for long stints. That's why exercises like a plank (and all the variations of it) are so great. In a standard plank, you have your toes and forearms on the floor, the belly button pulled in tight, neutral spine, and just hold. I encourage you to look online at how to perfect your form in a plank. This isometric exercise is great for building strength and endurance in your core muscles. It

Ideally, a strong core would allow you to sit upright without fatigue, walk tall for miles on end, and engage in sports with power to your limbs in all directions.

can be regressed for beginners (arms up on the wall or a bed) and progressed for the more advanced (feet elevated or a limb lifted). The goal is to feel the real work in your belly, not your lower back. I find it helpful to have my clients squeeze their

171

tush here as it forces a little pelvic tuck. This elongates the lower back and allows the lower belly muscles to engage.

You can do similar work for all the muscles on the back side of your trunk too. Quite often we forget that the "core" also includes your rear end and sides of the body. One of my favorite exercises for training the posterior core muscles is the bridge. You just lay on your back with your knees bent and feet on the floor. From there, you lift your hips up off the ground, engaging your tush and back muscles. I also like to have my clients press their shoulders into the floor to get the upper back firing up. If getting on the floor is not an option for you, you can do this in the comfort of your bed. You can see the bridge demonstrated on page [tbd].

Isometric exercises should be held for as long as you can with both good form and proper breathing. Make sure you are not holding your breath and that you can have an easy conversation while doing them. Start with just a few seconds' hold if that's where you are at. Try working your way up to one minute for each. When that comes more naturally, you can progress the exercise to make it slightly more challenging. Fun "core" exercises like crunches, sit-ups, and leg drops, are fine and can help you even get a more defined look in your abdominal muscles, but if you are not incorporating isometrics into your core workout routine, you are really missing the boat! Just know that if you don't have really good basic core strength and endurance (i.e., isometrics as described above), you still won't have a strong core. Sure, you may look good in a bikini or with your shirt off, but your posture won't be able to sustain itself.

Think about the confidence that you can exude when you stand tall—alpha even. We all know that person who, regardless of the situation, seems to always be standing with strength. Their chin is lifted, shoulders down and back, feet planted, eyes wide. These people command your attention. They don't cower or try to make themselves small. When they walk into a room, you know they are there.

Isometric exercises should be held for as long as you can with both good form and proper breathing.

They want you to know they are there. They might not even be cocky—they are just confident. And it all comes from how they hold their posture.

One of my favorite takeaways from a wonderful resource I read years ago (*Becoming a Supple Leopard* by Dr. Kelly Starrett) was the concept of "screwing in and stacking up." I have used this with hundreds of clients over the years, myself included. The whole book helps you understand the interconnectedness of your whole body: soft tissues rely on each other for proper movement. When it comes to setting your posture, you have to start from the ground up. Stand with your feet about hip-width apart, barefoot, and all ten toes facing straight ahead. Spread your toes as wide as you can and think about grabbing the floor with them. Then "screw" your legs into the ground. That means, without moving your feet at all, externally rotate your upper legs/femurs, which requires you to squeeze your bum. Not a lot, just enough that you can tell your butt is actively engaged. From here, you just make a little space between your hip bones and rib cage by sliding your rib cage and shoulders in perfect alignment over your hips. You may feel like you're leaning back a bit, but you are not. Your abdominals will naturally feel engaged. Then you slide your head in line with your shoulders. Not chin up, but just directly over your shoulders.

Going from a slumped-over, caved-in position to a taller, broader, and almost alpha stance makes a big difference in how you present yourself to the world as well as how you perceive yourself. Not only that, but with all of your core muscles appropriately working, and your limbs having a good base to work off of, you will be able to sustain this for long periods of time. You can also find examples of how to keep this alignment in Esther Gokhale's book, *8 Steps to a Pain-Free Back*. She shows you how humans have evolved to hold good posture throughout the day in all types of movement. From walking to sitting to standing, we have all the muscles and ability to keep ideal posture throughout the day; we just have to be aware and practice.

Changing It Up

We've had this conversation before, and I have to bring it up again. Remember, you are that amazing dynamic creature that is constantly evolving. The only constant your body will give you is change. Once you've been working through your workouts as we lined up above for a while, you may notice that you stop seeing results. Maybe you are doing too much HIIT and too little strength training. Maybe you are tighter than before and need to get more regular stretching in. Regardless, that is when you go back to the beginning of the "Move" chapter and start reassessing your current routines. Ask yourself, "Have my goals changed?" and "Why do I want to achieve those goals?" Then you can figure out what needs tweaking. And don't forget, this is also a great time to look at your nourishment too. It might be a good time to flip back to those pages and do some tweaking.

CHAPTER THREE

Explore

The next major component of "owning your wellness" is exploring. This section will *explore* what other healing and wellness opportunities you have yet to uncover. How do you know that the changes you have made are working for you? How do you know when those changes are no longer working? What are your symptoms possibly telling you? What have you not tried yet? This is what I mean by "explore." Maybe you need to do stool testing, hormone testing, or basic blood work to see what is happening inside. Lab testing helps you truly put all the health advice out there into the unique context of *you*.

One of the main things I do with my health coaching clients is assess, reassess, and often course correct what we are doing.

Exploring where you are, where you have been, and where you need to go is where my guidance differs greatly from other health and wellness books. *One of the main things I do with my health coaching clients is assess, reassess, and often course correct what we are doing.* What worked for weight loss in your twenties might not work at all in your fifties. And what works for your best friend might be horrific for you. Peer pressure and keeping up with the Joneses just don't work when it comes to evaluating what changes you should make (or not make) to feel your best.

As I settle into my midforties, I wish I could go back and tell my teen or twenties me, "Listen to your gut, girl!" Good Lord, I would have saved myself *so* many headaches and hard lessons if I had only just gone with my gut. This is true on the grander scale (dudes I should have never given my phone number to) and the smaller scale (not having that extra cocktail).

> Not only do the brain and belly talk about feelings, but they talk about other things like your overall health.

What I didn't understand was that my brain and gut actually talk to each other all the time. The gut-brain connection is strong! You know that feeling of butterflies in your tummy when you are super excited? Or that wave of nausea that hits when you learn of something really shocking or stressful? That is your brain and gut having a conversation.

The mind and gut send signals back and forth via the vagus nerve.[11] This nerve is the reason that you can't eat when you are depressed or only want to eat when you are nervous. **Not only do the brain and belly talk about feelings, but they talk about other things like your overall health.** When the gut tells the brain, "Hey, things aren't looking good down here," your brain gets the signal it might be time to get you to rest. In fact, your gut holds the key to your immune system! If your gut is healthy and full of happy, robust microbiota, the rest of you is likely feeling pretty good too. But when your gut is struggling to digest the wrong kind of foods (for you) or is riddled with inflammation from stress, the rest of you feels pretty crappy too.

Some people develop a bit of a disconnect between the brain and gut; they don't have very good conduction via the vagus nerve. There are many ways you can stimulate this nerve to increase its tone and strength. Things like gargling, humming, singing, chanting, and even laughing all increase vagal tone. Think about it this way, have you ever been a stress case trying to figure out a way to get the heck out of a gnarly situation and then suddenly burst into song?! No! When we sing along to our favorite tune or hum our way through doing chores, we are generally in a pretty chill state of mind. Your body equates that action of humming, singing, and so on, to being safe and well. *If you want to do just one thing to help yourself feel better on a daily basis, start piping up in the shower or while you are driving in the car.*

> # If you want to do just one thing to help yourself feel better on a daily basis, start piping up in the shower or while you are driving in the car.

Look for the Signals

One of the many things I help my clients with is getting in tune with the signals the body gives them. If you take time and pay attention, you'll find that there are many clues (some not so subtle) that your body is sending you about your health. While the list below is hardly exhaustive, it includes some pretty important symptoms to take note of.

Poop

From how frequently you go to what it looks and smells like, your poop is a good indicator of many things: whether you're eating the right foods (again, for *you*), whether you have the right mix of healthy gut bugs (microbiota), whether you're handling stress well, and even whether you're drinking enough water. While everyone is slightly different in cadence and quantity when it comes to BMs, there are some basics to look for. ***Ideally, you should go every day.*** Yes, ladies, I'm talking to you. Once or twice a week is not cutting it. Even if that is how often you have always gone, it's not enough. When stool stays in the colon for too long, we run the risk of toxins getting recirculated into the bloodstream. Going #2 at least once per day ensures that your transit time (the time it takes for food to go from one end to get out the other) isn't too long. Your poop not only contains fiber and undigested bits of food but also is one of the main ways you detoxify other things like hormones and environmental toxins.

If your poop is hard (constipation) or too runny (diarrhea), you have another indicator that something is not right. One of the main culprits in constipation is dehydration. Your colon will need enough water to absorb and make stool easier to push out. Yes, you might need more fiber, but make sure you also get plenty of water. Reminder: your morning "inner bath," wink, wink. If you are struggling with diarrhea on a regular basis, you might need to look at food sensitivities. Clearly, you are eating something(s) that are just not digested well by your gut. It could also be that you are getting too much roughage for your system, and it might be time to pull back on the giant salads for dinner. I find that I can have one great big serving of veggies in a day, but two is way too many!

Runny and/or floating poops are an indication that you are not digesting fats very well or that you are having too much fat in your diet. You might want to consider some digestive enzymes with lipases and proteases (enzymes for fats and proteins) to take with meals. Conversely, if yours are dry and harder to get out, you might need a bit more fat, fiber, or both.

Lastly, it should not stink! Yes, there may be a little odor, but if you have to warn the household not to come within twenty feet of the bathroom for a while, you have a problem.

Basically, your shit should not stink!

Likely, you are, again, eating something that is not well-digested or is fermenting in your gut. Keep in mind we are not like cows or gorillas that have multiple stomach chambers. We are not designed to digest copious amounts of vegetation all day long. If you notice bloating, gassiness, and stinky poos, you need to reassess what your meals look like. ***Basically, your shit should not stink!***

Skin

Your skin is the largest organ you have. It is also the first line of defense against the world around us. Only certain things should get through it in either direction. When you meet someone who has glowing, clear skin, what do you think? I immediately think, "Wow, that person looks so healthy!" And

Like it or not, our skin signals to those around us how healthy we are.

what about when you meet someone who looks sallow, blemished, and blotchy? I think, "They need to get some sun, exercise, and water." ***Like it or not, our skin signals to those around us how healthy we are.*** And if you pay attention to yours, it is giving you good signals too.

For most of my adolescence and early adult life, I had horrible "chicken skin" on my thighs and the backs of my arms. I just thought it was that I didn't exfoliate enough or that I needed better lotion. But nothing seemed to make it better. Then, I gave up dairy. Within about two weeks, my skin cleared up. I mean smooth as can be. It was crazy! Then, about a year later, I started getting it back. I realized that the protein bars I was eating had whey protein in them (a dairy protein). I got rid of them, and wham! No more chicken skin.

I'm telling you, figure out what is happening inside of you to cause the symptoms you notice on the outside!

I'm not saying you have to give up dairy to have clear skin, but you do need to look at the signs your skin is giving you. Do you have eczema? If so, this too might be a food sensitivity issue. In fact, both my daughter and I avoid wheat like the plague. Just one erroneous bite will leave us with patches of eczema along our arms, back, and belly. *I'm telling you, figure out what is happening inside of you to cause the symptoms you notice on the outside!*

No conversation about skin health would be complete without a mention of pimples. The type of pimples and the location of pimples can tell you a lot about what is going on inside of your body. When we were kids, my brother and I both had acne: his on his face and mine on my shoulders. He was told he just didn't wash well enough and ate too much pizza and sugar. I was told to pull my hair up. I now know that both of us were just dealing with acne due to huge swings in our hormones. His testosterone surges and my estrogen/progesterone cycles were sputtering their way along, and our skin was just telling the tale. We both made the mistake of listening to the dogma of the time and putting gallons of SeaBreeze and Oxy on ourselves, which only stripped the skin of the oils it needed and made matters worse.

Men, if you are getting pimples on your back or shoulders, chances are you are having some hormone dysregulation. Ladies, if you are getting pimples at the same time every month, the same goes for you. Also, if your pimples are cystic: you know, those deep painful ones that are so buried so deep into you it looks like you're growing another eye! Yeah, those. If you suffer from cystic acne (male, female, or anything in between), get your hormones checked![12] Note: more details are coming on this testing later in the "Explore" chapter.

Let's also chat briefly about autoimmune conditions that show up on the skin. Psoriasis, dandruff, alopecia, and so on, are all conditions where your body's own immune system thinks that those skin cells are foreign invaders and attack them. While autoimmunity issues are often genetic, they don't have to overrun your life. By working on nourishing yourself well, moving the right amount, and getting your gut and immune system strong, you can quell the intensity of these autoimmune symptoms. I encourage you to do some research on healing "leaky gut" and even consider working with someone like myself or a functional/integrative doctor to help guide you toward calming autoimmunity. You can also do a quick Amazon search for the "autoimmune protocol," and you'll see that you are not alone and have many resources at your disposal. In the case of psoriasis, there often is an issue with other detoxifying organs not doing their jobs so well. When the liver and/or kidneys aren't able to keep up, the skin then tries to take over the detoxification burden.[13] This will only exacerbate the underlying psoriatic issue. If psoriatic plaques, dandruff, eczema, and so on, are issues you struggle with, it's time for you to listen to the clues your skin is giving you and get to the root of the issue.

Sweat

While we are on the topic of skin, let's talk about how it breathes. Some people are seriously sweaty, while others barely get dewy upon exertion. Regardless of where you fall on the sweaty spectrum, your body also gives you clues about your health through your sweat. Over- or undersweating can tell you if your autonomic system can cool itself appropriately and if you have good circulation. Knowing if you have really stinky sweat can tell you if maybe there is a toxic burden on your body and you could use some detox help. And if you are the kind of person who has really salty sweat, you may be in danger of dehydration more than others.

First of all, does your sweat stink? Granted, most of us will smell from being sweaty if we let it dry on us and don't shower or change clothes. But if your sweat smells from the onset, you need to pay attention to what your lymphatic system is doing. Your body is either moving toxins through you that are problematic or you are not able to detoxify well. Take a look at your medications, your food choices, and of course, your body products. Keep in mind that transdermal application (through the skin) is one of the most effective ways to get medication into someone's bloodstream. However, for that exact reason, we have to be careful what we put *on* our skin because it too will get through our pores and into circulation. Make sure your skincare products are not laden with chemicals that are toxic to you.

If you find that you have a really hard time breaking a sweat, no matter how hot it is or how hard you are working, you may be struggling with hypohidrosis. This can actually be a serious medical issue, as it affects how your body can cool itself.[14] I struggle a bit with this myself but have found ways to make it better. In fact, I get so overheated (and conversely freeze when it's too cold) that I basically try to live where it is always between 60 and 80°. But what I didn't realize is that this lack of sweating is actually tied to a general issue with my circulation. I suffer from varicose veins, Raynaud's phenomenon (where my fingertips and toes turn white-numb when cold), and even chilblains. That last one is a doozy: when I get too cold for too long, then try to warm my toes and fingers up, they can get inflammation trapped in them, and I end up with little ulcers on my digits that take months to heal. Fun!

I tell you all this because that one symptom (not sweating readily) was quite the canary in the coal mine when it came to other health issues. It was a clue that my circulation was bad. When tied together with my varicose and spider veins in my teen years, then all the other symptoms that popped up, my body was giving me *huge* signals: hey, you need to work on this!

Aches and Pains

How many of you just trump up achy joints and niggling pains to age? Or do you get frequent headaches or migraines and just think that's normal for you? ***Believe it or not, hurting does not have to be part of aging.*** Pain is just another (rather loud) signal from your body that something is wrong. In my late twenties, I had really bad pain in my right shoulder that was so frustrating. When I went to the doctor, he sent me to an orthopedic specialist, who assured me that rotator cuff surgery was the only option. "Really?" I thought.

> Believe it or not, hurting does not have to be part of aging.

"How is that possible?" Well, he was really, really wrong. I just had some faulty movement patterns and not-so-great posture, and I needed to work on my upper back strength. Oh, and a few massages helped too. If I had been in my sixties, not my twenties, I might have just said, "Doc, I'm sure you're right. Let's do it." What a waste that would have been.

That's not to say that surgery doesn't have its place, but only when it is truly medically necessary. If you have aches or pains that are just sort of nagging annoyances, look deeper. One of the many signals I got from my body that I wasn't giving it the right mix of nourishing food and movement was chronic pain under my kneecaps. This is a very common issue with runners and is thought of as being unavoidable. You'll hear that you just need to stretch your IT bands and hips, warm up more, and maybe try some physical therapy. I did all those things and thought that years of pounding the pavement, downhill skiing, and dancing had just done me in. But when I totally cleaned up my diet, and when I got on the Paleo bandwagon around 2010, that once chronic knee pain just disappeared. Gone.

It's funny how it can take a while to notice a lack of pain. It was probably a couple of months before I thought to myself, "Wow, I don't even think about my knees anymore!" It just sort of happened. The funny thing is that every once in a blue moon, I get a little ache under those kneecaps again. Yes, sometimes it's because I had a hard workout or haven't been keeping up with my yoga. But often, it's when I've been recklessly noshing on things like dairy and gluten, and I take it as my body's not-so-subtle reminder that it's time to get my butt back in line!

Hunger and Cravings

I could write a whole chapter on how your hunger pangs and specific cravings can give insights into your overall health. *Though many of us no longer trust them, our bodies really do know what they need and will send signals in the form of cravings and tummy grumbles to ask for it.* For example, if you wake up in the middle of the night and feel the need to have a snack, you are dealing with some blood sugar issues. Same thing if you wake up in the morning starving. If you find yourself craving salty and crunchy foods, your adrenal glands are probably asking you for some much-needed salt and other minerals to help them function better. Craving chocolate during PMS? You probably need some magnesium, which is a rather calming mineral.

The first time I remember really

Though many of us no longer trust them, our bodies really do know what they need and will send signals in the form of cravings and tummy grumbles to ask for it.

189

noticing how hunger and cravings were actually my body asking for specific nutrients was when I was pregnant. I had these insatiable urges for avocados and blueberries. Not things I generally ever wanted before. But my little one was sending signals to my body that it needed lots of healthy fats to grow that brain of hers, and plenty of antioxidants to keep her thriving.

Now, clearly every niggling yen for a goody is not necessarily tied to a true physiological need. In fact, if you have gotten in the habit of noshing on the wrong things for your health and goals for too long, you may find that you are having cravings for all kinds of things you know are not good for you. For example, if you wake up hungry and immediately reach for a vanilla latte to go with your bowl of cereal or bagel, chances are you are going to crave more and more sugar all day long. If this sounds familiar, please go back to the "Nourish" chapter and reread the first few sections.

Sleep

This is another signal that is worthy of a whole tome. In fact, there are many amazing books on the subject, one of my favorites being *Sleep Smarter* by Shawn Stevenson. If you want more details, tips, and tricks, go check it out. ***But know that your sleep quality and quantity can tell you a lot about what is going on inside your mind and body.***

If you wake up in a puddle of sweat, chances are there is

some hormone dysregulation going on. Note this is not just a problem for women in menopause. This issue can be problematic for those with hyperthyroidism, insufficient progesterone, and blood sugar issues. In fact, going to bed with too much sugar in your system (either from food or alcohol) can often lead to hypoglycemia in the middle of the night. Once your body finally processes all that sugar, your levels drop so low that your body then shoots up your cortisol (stress hormone) to try to get more sugar flowing into your blood again. This will wake you up so fast! Have you ever been out having maybe one or two too many cocktails, come home to pass out immediately, then shot up at like 2 a.m.? Well, now you know why.

But know that your sleep quality and quantity can tell you a lot about what is going on inside your mind and body.

If you are having a hard time falling asleep, chances are you are getting to bed with too much of the stress hormone cortisol still flowing through you and maybe not enough melatonin to help you get ready to snooze. This signal is telling you that you need to bring down the intensity a couple of hours before bed. By disengaging from work, personal stress, and electronics, you might be able to calm that spinning mind of yours to fall asleep sooner. You may also not be getting enough sunshine during the day. Keep in mind, your brain is still functioning off a millennia-old operating system. I keep waiting for the cosmos to shoot up a system upgrade, but no luck so far. We need the sun (from sunrise through midday and sunset) to signal to our brains what time it is and when to sleep. If you are stuck inside looking at fake lights from your devices, your poor old-school brain just won't believe you when it's time to finally get some shut-eye.

And if you are the type of person who just wakes up all through the night and can't stay down, you likely have a combination of all the things above going on. Whatever your issue with sleep is, take note of it and spend some time figuring out why. Even if it's been an issue for you all your life, that doesn't mean it's okay. It means that you should get going on fixing the problem ASAP. Sleep is key for so many reasons, so don't poo-poo this one!

Mood

This one is tricky but worth discussing. While we all have some moodiness here and there, being the kind of person who is high and then low all the time is not ideal. I'm not judging you if your claim to infamy is your saucy biting tongue, but just know that your hot/cold temperament might be an indicator that something else is going on with you.

Remember our conversation about the gut-brain connection? Sometimes having feelings of depression, anxiety, or even mania can be related to the health of your gut. In fact, some not-so-great gut bugs are directly correlated with specific mood disorders. When I first got involved with the functional health world, I was going through a separation. The stress was so intense that my insides were trying to run for the hills. I was a mess. I decided to do a stool test to see what was going on in there. Turns out that one of the nasty parasites that was proliferating in my gut, Cryptosporidium, is often found in those with anorexia nervosa. My head exploded! How long had I had this? Disordered eating had been an issue for me for many years at this point, and could it be that this darn parasitic infection was at the root? While it may have been somewhat dormant in my gut for a while, the stress of my separation allowed that darn Crypto to go unchecked and rear its ugly head again.

Of course, not all mood issues are related just to your gut (though it's always intertwined). Often there is a hormonal element as well. From sex hormones to thyroid and adrenal hormones, your mood and its steadiness are very much dependent on all these things to be humming along well. And, of course, there's sleep. Not only can your mood be affected by the quality and quantity of your sleep but your mood can affect that quality and quantity of your sleep right back!

If your friends and family tell you all too often what kind of mood they are picking up on, try your best not to get offended. Though a good snap-back here and there will definitely keep them in line. Then spend some time thinking about what might be going on with you that could be causing the Dr. Jekyll and Mr. Hyde situation.

Cognition

How quickly your mind works, how well you can retrieve and retain information, and how easily you problem-solve are all great indications of how healthy your brain is. ***Don't get fooled into thinking senility is just a function of age.*** Just because memory loss and word retrieval issues are common doesn't mean you have to just accept them as part of your life. If you have noticed a decline in your once-quick processing speed, it is a strong signal that there is some underlying inflammation or other cause that needs your attention.

> Don't get fooled into thinking senility is just a function of age.

The term "leaky gut" refers to the tight junctions between the cells lining your small intestine being loosened. This can then lead to particles getting into your bloodstream that may be toxic or inflammatory. This same issue can happen to your brain. There is a tightly regulated seal around our brains called the "blood-brain barrier." Only the nutrients that our brains need to thrive should be let through. However, with stress, toxic exposures, consumption of inflammatory foods, and so on. (all things that also cause leaky gut), that blood-brain barrier can become more porous than is ideal. This means that our precious noggins aren't as well protected as they should be.

When there is inflammation in our brains, their function gets impaired. You may notice this in the form of how fast you process information, how well you retain or retrieve information, or even how you move. If there are noticeable deficits for you, take stock of what might be causing this. Are you inflamed in other parts of your body: gut, skin, joints?

You could also consider looking at heavy metal or mold exposure. How are you managing the stressors in your life? Are you eating foods that might not be working for you anymore? Are you taking medications that impact your gut health? Remember, the gut and brain are sympatico. If one is not feeling well, neither is the other!

Libido

I'm going to try to avoid the minefield here and just keep my comments general. While, of course, there are a million reasons why you may not be "in the mood," if that is your every day, you might want to evaluate why. Aside from not having a partner that makes your knees weak, a lack of libido can also be a sign of some underlying health issues. Being overweight, especially around your middle, can indicate that you have too much estrogen (or testosterone being converted to estrogen). In both men and women, excess estrogen can wreak havoc on your health in lots of ways, but libido can be collateral damage. Stress overload is also never good on your yen for lovin' either. If either of these is a possible reason for your lack of libido (overweight and/or stress), you might consider getting your hormones checked. Learning about how your body is producing and detoxifying hormones like estrogen, testosterone, progesterone, cortisol, and DHEA can give you amazing clues on how to feel better globally.

Now Let's Connect the Dots

What if, in reading the above possible signals your body is giving you, you identify with several? This is where we continue our exploration of what is going on and, more importantly, why. For example, let's say you are having foggy thinking almost every afternoon, have digestive issues a few times a week, and have nagging eczema that never seems to clear up. In that case, you might want to work with a practitioner to test your stool to see what kind of gut bugs (good and not so good) you have. You may also look for food sensitivities or allergies. This is where working with a really good functional medicine doctor or functional health coach can be a game changer. But even if you find someone amazing, you need to know what questions to ask and why. Being not only interested but involved in your own testing, results, and treatment plans is critical to your long-term health success.

I will show you plenty of ways below to do some detective

work on your own. However, if things get a little tricky, you might consider reaching out to get a good health professional on your team. Here are some websites to get you started in that search:

For guidance along your health journey, you can find a functional diagnostic nutrition health coach, like me, at FDN Thrive: https://fdnthrive.com.

For a functional medicine doctor near you, do a search at the Institute for Functional Medicine: https://www.ifm.org/find-a-practitioner/.

Before we move on, let's not lose sight of all that we just learned. Below, take a moment to jot down any symptoms or signs for each category that popped up for you. You will want to have these fresh in your head as we work on figuring out *why* those signals are trying to get your attention:

	Possible Symptoms /Signals	Possible Reasons Why the Symptom or Signal Is Happening
Poop		
Skin		
Sweat		
Aches		
Hunger		
Sleep		
Mood		
Cognition		
Libido		

Know Where You've Been, Where You Are, and Where You Are Going

Whether you made notes in each category above or only one, your body is sending you a clear sign that something is wrong. If a red light popped up on your car's dashboard, you wouldn't ignore it for very long. The notes you made in the chart are your body's red lights! Don't ignore them. While you may be able to replace your car, you cannot replace your body. Why would you pay less heed to its maintenance needs?

Don't wait. Start now.
Don't wait. Start now.
Don't wait. Start now.

There is no other way to say it. There is no magical date on the calendar that is going to make the changes any easier. There is no point in time in the future when life is going to suddenly be simpler and starting a new program will be just perfect. The more you wait, the more you lose sight of how important those changes are. Just like you can't keep driving on a flat tire for very long, you can't ignore the pain in your back (or the horrible digestive issues, or even the foggy thinking) for very long before your system just won't go anymore. Don't get stranded on the side of the road, folks. Fix it now. Okay, enough with the car analogy. While I am far from perfect on this, I do a pretty good job at making the serious changes I need to make today. Not tomorrow. Not next week. Not the first of the year. Now. If I know that _____ is problematic for my health and happiness or for that of my family, it starts now.

Not only does "it" need to start now but obviously we need to know what "it" is. Let's go back and look at the chart above. Which symptom is the most frustrating, life-affecting, or even just the most annoying? Put that one at the top of the list. If being in a crappy mood more days than not is affecting your quality of life because no one wants to be around you, you better fix that ASAP! And yes, you may have some digestive issues and low libido too, but you decide that mood is the first priority to work on. Good. Once you know that, the detective work begins. And don't think that the tummy and sexy-time trouble won't be addressed. Chances are, those other issues will be intricately entwined with the mood issue. *Start working on just one, and you'll be surprised to see how the other issues either resolve too or at least start improving.*

> Start working on just one, and you'll be surprised to see how the other issues either resolve too or at least start improving.

Where You Are

Once you figure out what the number one issue is you're going to start working on, you can then begin figuring out where you are starting from. This can be as simple as using the workbook pages in this book to take notes on what is going on with you. You can also use a personal journal or even just a new note on your smartphone. Write down all the things related to that one issue. I find that allowing myself to pour out a stream of consciousness on paper helps me start getting some clues. In keeping with our crappy mood example from above, maybe you jot down notes like:

- *Mornings are really hard.*

- *Sleeping in somehow makes it worse.*

- *This seems to have started a few months ago.*

- *What happened a few months ago? OMG— my dog died around then.*

- *I stopped going for walks with him.*

- *I actually feel a little better when I go outside to eat my lunch.*

- *I'm also really bored at night lately.*

- *I don't have that much fun stuff to look forward to.*

- *I just sit at home and watch Netflix.*

- *Sometimes I'm up way later than I should be because I get hooked watching something.*

- *Then I sleep in too late.*

- *Then I feel crappier the next day.*

- *Oh, and my PMS has been really horrible lately.*

- *Like really bad.*

- *Wait, it wasn't always like that.*

- *It's worse since I gained those ten pounds.*

- *Which also creeped up on me after my dog passed.*

- *Do I need a new dog?*

- *Maybe I just need to go for a walk every day.*

You get the idea. So you sit down and let it flow. Then come back an hour later and read it. What jumps out at you? As a health coach, here's what I get from that:

- Possible vitamin D deficiency due to too much time inside and mood issues

- Some blood sugar dysregulation, either from diet or from lack of exercise or both

- Some sex hormone and stress hormone issues due to PMS

- Lack of human/animal interaction is causing a feeling of isolation

- Maybe some need for more protein and even minerals to help with sleep quality

- Too much exposure to blue light from devices in the evening is disrupting circadian rhythm.

Now, you might not have picked up on all of those things. Heck, you might have picked up several more. But do you see now how the one signal is actually part of all the other issues this person is dealing with?

If you'd like to use the space below to start your own rambling thoughts on what is going on with you, go for it:

_____

_____

_____

_____

_____

_____

_____

_____

_____

Where You Have Been

This may sound backward, but I think it's better to know where you are now before you compare it to where you've been. Are the things that came up for you as you discussed your problem things that have been of issue all along? Or are they new? In our example above, we see that this person gained ten pounds, stopped sleeping well, got bad PMS, and then ended up globally grumpy all since the time her dog passed away. That's not to say that the dog is the issue necessarily, but at least she can see that she didn't always feel this way.

What if she did? What if your main issue right now is something that you have struggled with your entire life? Just because it isn't new doesn't mean that you're stuck dealing with it forever. I had that darn eczema and chicken skin on my arms and legs for as long as I could remember. But when I did a little detective work and figured out the trigger for those skin issues, I was surprised and relieved that I didn't have to go on hiding those rough spots. You may not find the "cure" for what ails you, but I bet you can find your own triggers and at least feel a heck of a lot better! ***You don't have to settle for just feeling mediocre. You can feel great!***

> You don't have to settle for just feeling mediocre. You can feel great!

Self-Quantifying

Once you know where you have been and where you are, you can start tracking your progress. Years ago, the concept of "self-quantifying" was all over the health blogosphere. It's a tech/fancy way of saying, "track your progress." Being in Silicon Valley in the late 20-aughts, it seemed like every want-to-be health-tech lover was running "n = 1" experiments on themselves. We all started tracking steps, sleep, calories consumed, calories burned, and on and on. That's all fine and well, but what do you do with all this data? The only reason to self-quantify is to know where you are starting, what progress you are making, and what sort of goal makes all those data points have value.

Track only what needs tracking. If you are a healthy weight/size and just want to work on flexibility, who cares how many steps you take in a day? If you are concerned about your waist size, then steps per day might matter. My point is, think about what your main concern is and find one or two data points you can easily measure and keep track of. Here are some examples that might help you get on the right path. In each row that lists an issue you are dealing with, go through the ideas I have given you for data to gather. Then, make some personal notes on the ones that make sense to you. I'm sure I've left out some options, so please insert your own if you have additional ideas.

Issue	Possible Quantifiable Data	Personal Notes
Diarrhea /constipation	-# of times/day or week you go and consistency -Meal eaten directly before diarrhea episode -Grams of fiber eaten per day -Ounces of water consumed daily	
Eczema	-Location and size of the patches -Pictures of said patches after removing one food group for a month -Improvement or not with changes to skin creams -Seasonality of it	
Stinky sweat	-Meals eaten prior to noticing smell -Ounces of water consumed daily -Changes after switching deodorant	
Chronic neck pain	-Changes when adjustments are made to computer setup -How many hours per day using gadgets -Improvements after massage or PT -Changes from new pillow or sleeping position	
Middle of the night hunger/ cravings	-Dinner preceding -Perceived stress level day before or impending -Temperature of room -Menstrual cycle phase -Seasonality -Blood sugar levels	
Hard time falling asleep	-Exposure to blue light in hours preceding bedtime -Caffeine intake and timing -Alcohol intake and timing -Quality and timing of dinner -Perceived stress -Exposure to nature/natural sunlight -Heart rate variability (HRV)	
Quick temper, even without provocation	-Blood sugar levels -Hormone levels -Quality and timing of meals prior -Menstrual cycles -Exposure to nature/natural sunlight	
Foggy thinking, especially in afternoon	-Lunch consumed prior -Caffeine consumption prior -Quality of sleep night before -Exposure to natural light -Exercise that day -Digestive issues	
Rarely any libido	-Recent blood work with information on cholesterol and sex hormones -Sleep quality on average -Changes in diet -Regular exercise	

Some of the above suggestions might leave you scratching your head. Like, why would tracking my digestive issues give me an idea of why I have foggy thinking? Well, that's because having bacteria or parasites in your small intestine can actually affect how well your brain is working! Now, keep in mind making those connections is my specialty. But I put together this list to get you thinking again about how one symptom you are noticing might actually be interconnected with all your other health issues.

Don't let yourself get overwhelmed. If all that sounds too complicated, and you're starting to glaze over, let's make this simple. ***Pick just* one *thing— one measurable, trackable thing— and start paying attention to that.*** It could be as simple as measuring your waist circumference. Just knowing that one data point can help you make better decisions toward getting that number down. If you measure your waist and realize you are ten inches away from your goal, you are not as likely to grab donuts for breakfast five minutes later. The sheer act of quantifying that single data point helps inform your decisions subconsciously.

Aside from helping my clients connect the dots, I also help them by being a built-in accountability buddy. Find someone who cares about your health to check in with. Tell them, "Hey, I just measured my waist, and I'm trying to lose ten inches in the next six months. Can I check in with you once a week and just let you know how I'm doing?" Not only will most good friends say, "Of course!" but many will be inspired to start their own health changes. Then you can check in and hold each other accountable for staying on task. Owning your wellness doesn't have to be a singular journey. Like most trips, it is much more fun with friends!

Pick just *one* thing— one measurable, trackable thing— and start paying attention.

Once you have the one thing you are going to start tracking and a friend to share your journey with, pick one thing you can change right now to get going in the right direction. If losing ten inches off your waist was your top priority, and you are using that tape measure weekly to stay on top of your progress, what will you do to reach that goal? Don't choose five things to change today. Choose one and make it a habit. Give yourself a week or two, or even a month, before you make the next change. Don't go keto, hire a trainer, start using new supplements, and join a run club all at once. How will you know what is working? Better yet, how will you know what is NOT working for you?

Maybe you hire a trainer and get a new workout routine going twice a week. After a month, you've lost two inches.

Then the following month, you try a lower-carb diet and stick with it for a few weeks. After three weeks, you see you've lost another inch and a half. Maybe you decide that's enough changes and let your body settle into a new groove. Then a month later, after the waistline stays about the same, you know it's time to layer in those morning jogs with your friends' group once a week. *Adding in changes gradually, scientifically even, allows you to see how you are impacting your progress toward your goal.*

> Adding in changes gradually, scientifically even, allows you to see how you are impacting your progress toward your goal.

Taking this more scientific method to introduce changes also allows you to see when a new piece just doesn't fit into your health puzzle. Maybe adding in the jogging actually causes you more stress, which in turn kicks up inflammation and causes you to gain weight in your waist! It happens; trust me! So you realize, keeping all things constant, if you switch those jogs to brisk walks with a good friend, you might feel less stressed. Getting some time with a buddy and the exercise that you need without the anxiety of having to ramp up to running might be a better solution for you.

You should also make note of changes you notice in other areas of your health. As your waistline starts to slim down, do you notice your afternoon energy perking up naturally? Do you find yourself more interested in cuddling up with your spouse? Are you waking up more refreshed in the morning? This is why it is so important to make some notes early on about how you feel as you begin your wellness journey. ***How will you know how far you've come if you don't know where you started?***

Stay steady, until you shouldn't . . . And don't give up! You will have hard days. You will make mistakes. You'll want to give up. You'll tell yourself you have to start over. DO NOT. Remember, this is not a flat road. Those speed bumps will slow you down. Do not let them stop you, though. They are just speed bumps. Stay the course. Try new things. Stop the stuff that doesn't work for you. Keep it simple. But don't stop.

While we are on the topic, eventually, some of the changes you are making now will no longer work for you. Maybe going low-carb at forty helped you lose and keep off twenty pounds. But suddenly, at fifty, those twenty pounds creep back on regardless of how few grams of carbohydrates

> # How will you know how far you've come if you don't know where you started?

you restrict to. In fact, this was exactly what happened to my husband. When he was in his early forties, he dropped to a zero-sugar, high-fat diet. He was running one hundred miles a month. He lifted three days a week. He went from about 250 pounds to 160 pounds of pure muscle. It wasn't easy, but it sure worked. Then, ten years later, the weight crept back up to around 200. The running, even though harder with the extra pounds, was not doing anything to keep his weight in check. He was still eating fewer carbs than about anyone I had met. But still, there he was, feeling frustrated to be carrying so much more weight despite his efforts.

He needed a change. What worked for his body's chemistry a decade ago was no longer going to do it. He started working with a new trainer who suggested he instead try to get more of his calories from veggies, try eating low-fat, and focus his workouts on weight training instead of cardio. Within six months, he dropped over thirty pounds. He was visibly laying down serious muscle. He not only looked great but felt great. The hours not being lost on running allowed him to manage work stress better too. And as great as all that is, he knows that at some point, these changes may stop working. It will be time to reassess.

You, too, may find that after a while, your diet or fitness regimen may need some adjustments. It's not that you're getting old. Gaining weight, getting achy, and having a hard time retrieving thoughts are not just a function of age. Make changes. Flip back to the "Nourish" and "Move" chapters to see how your goals and "why" have changed. Then make one (just one) adjustment. Just try one different thing and give it a month or so. See if that moves the needle a bit. If it does, great, stick with it and then maybe layer in one or two more changes (one at a time). But if that first tweak you chose doesn't work, don't get frustrated. Try something else.

Have a little patience with yourself. Your body endures a lot, so be nice to it. Be nice to you. Just because you may not fit into those old skinny jeans anymore doesn't mean you won't again—or better yet, that you should! Maybe you need to readjust what matters. Can you love who and what you see, even if you know you could be healthier? *You and your body are on the same team.* This was a really hard lesson for me to learn. Yes, I will always strive to be healthier, live longer, and have even more energy. But being kind to myself for not being perfect has taken me decades. Try looking at yourself in the mirror without judging what you see. You

You and your body are on the same team.

are seeing you. You are a remarkable person. I don't know you, but I know that! Do you think your family looks at you and sees all the wrinkles on your face or the cellulite on your thighs? Nope. They just see you. Care for yourself; no one else will if you don't.

Testing Takes the Guesswork Out

So you've spent a fair amount of time and energy assessing what signals your body may be giving you. You've made adjustments to your nutrition, exercise, rest, and stress management. And yet maybe you still aren't feeling like you're on the right path toward reaching your goals. This is the point where some additional testing might be warranted.

"Test, don't guess." The founder of FDN where I studied, Reed Davis, has lots of little catch phrases. My favorite one by far is, *"Test, don't guess."* I even have a T-shirt with it written across the front. It should be the standard for each and every practitioner. Before you start tossing handfuls of supplements down your throat, test. Before you take an antibiotic (again), test. Before you sign up for some drug that you'll likely be on for the rest of your life, test!

Whether you're concerned about hormones, inflammation, allergies, food sensitivities, bone density, or just general health, it's a good idea to have some data points to work off of. I will explain a few of my favorite test options below. These are by no means a complete list of options. However, keep in mind that the main value in testing at all is *what you will do with the information.* Before you sign yourself up for any testing, ask yourself (or your practitioner), "What will I do with the results?" If you find out that you are highly reactive to many foods you love, will you be able to eliminate them? If you see that you are having digestive issues because of leaky gut and dysbiosis, will you be willing to go through the protocols your practitioner recommends to heal your gut? Just do a little check-in with yourself as you read through some of the testing I suggest below. What would knowing your results do for you?

Keep in mind, you have to put those results in the context of you!

It is critical that whomever you are working with doesn't look at your lab work only. The only actionable results should be the ones that clearly correlate with how you feel. You (or your health practitioner) should not be treating results; the treatment plan should be about you. Once you have lab work that you know makes sense in relation to your symptoms, then (and only then) can you work with your health coach to put together a game plan. I like to line up a ninety-day protocol to help my clients see the clear path in front of them. We take their results and then discuss how we are going to make adjustments to their nourishment, movement, lifestyle, and even supplements.

Again, I am not a doctor. I can order testing, help with organizing supplement protocols, and give my clients tons of research and support information to help them. However, there are times I need to refer out. I know what I know; I know what I don't know; I know when to research; and I know when to ask for help. I tell you this because you, too, should know when to ask for help. Yes, you can look at a lot of these tests yourself and do research on what to do with the results, but please seek additional assistance. Find a well-educated set of eyes to look at your health with you and help you formulate a plan. When I order testing for myself, I take it to my doctor to review. I need guidance and an objective point of view. So do you.

Possible Testing to Consider

While each of the testing options below focuses on specific issues and symptoms, you may also consider doing a combination of them. Rarely does just one test illuminate all that is going on for a client. For example, if chronic stress is at the root of their health issues, they may have a wonky cortisol pattern, some troublesome gut bugs, and be dealing with nutrient deficiencies. If a woman is having a bumpy time getting through menopause, she may also have a deficiency and/or overproduction of other hormones coinciding with some circulation issues that are impacting her body's ability to detoxify regularly, and she's very likely not having good digestion on top of it all. These are just examples of why it might be more effective (time and cost-wise) to run multiple tests at once and get all the information possible to get started on a good path to regaining wellness. That said, here are some additional details on specifics. Note, I do not delve into heavy metal screenings, nor mold testing. I have not been versed in either as of yet. In addition, you can garner much of this information from the organic acids testing mentioned below.

Basic Blood Panel

Just like with nourishment and movement, I like to start with the low-hanging fruit when it comes to any kind of testing. It's a good idea to get a yearly physical from your general practitioner. If you don't already do this or even have a GP, please take the time to do so. Having a good relationship with a Western medical doctor you trust is important. And make sure they get you in for a yearly check-up. Aside from an in-person visit to look at your vitals and discuss your current health concerns, they should also order a complete blood panel for you.

I often ask my clients to share with me a copy of their most recent blood panel, because from there, I can learn a lot about what is going on inside. First of all, keep in mind that your test results will be compared to the "standard lab ranges" determined by whichever lab is processing your blood draw. *This does not mean that they are comparing your results to those of a healthy person, but instead against the averages or means of all the people they are testing.*[15] While this doesn't apply to every data point on a standard panel, it applies to many. I don't know about you, but I do not want

This does not mean that they are comparing your results to those of a healthy person, but instead against the averages or means of all the people they are testing.

my health metrics graded on a scale that uses the average American. The average American is sick! Obesity, hypertension, diabetes, and heart disease are prevalent in our society. So keep that in mind when you see your results next to an expected range.

When I look at my own blood work or that of my clients, I compare those results to functional health ranges. These are numbers that are expected for optimal health in a person, not mediocrity. For example, one of the test results you may get back from your standard blood work is a *fasting glucose* number. Western medicine says that anything at or below 99 mg/dL is fine.[16] NO! If you are fasting for twelve hours and wake up with a blood sugar of 99, just thinking about breakfast will put you in pre-diabetic ranges. Instead, I like to see clients with fasting blood sugars of 90 mg/dL and under. If you are curious about how to compare your own blood panel results to those of healthy humans, you can do an internet search for "functional blood chemistry analysis" or look for an FDN or integrative health practitioner to help you.

The great thing about getting basic blood work done with your GP is that you will likely be able to get insurance to pay most of the cost. However, to make it personalized a bit more for you, it would be good to ask your doctor to include a few data points they might not otherwise think of. Depending on your family's medical history or your individual concerns, these might include the following:

- Fasting insulin: In conjunction with fasting blood sugar and a Hemoglobin A1C (average blood sugar over the last three months), this will give you a more complete picture of how your body is managing blood sugar and if you are in any danger of developing diabetes.[17]

- Advanced lipid screening: In addition to your standard cholesterol and triglyceride numbers, you may want to ask for additional data on your apolipoprotein B (ApoB) as well as your LDL particle count (LDL-P).[18] These can help give you better insights into your actual risk of developing cardiovascular disease. The less your ApoB and LDL-P, the healthier your circulating cholesterol numbers are.

- Thyroid: Sometimes (though not always), your doctor will order a single thyroid marker, TSH. Thyroid-stimulating hormone is a measure of how loud the signal is from your brain to your thyroid hormone to pump out more. The louder the signal, the more your thyroid is struggling. Optimal health ranges suggest this number to be between 0.5 and 2.5.[19] However, this is only a small part of the thyroid picture. You may want to request a few additional thyroid markers:[20]

- Free T4: thyroid hormone produced by your thyroid gland and available for use (should be in the upper ⅓ of lab ranges)

- Free T3: the more active form of thyroid hormone converted from T4 (should also be in the upper ⅓ of lab ranges)

- Reverse T3: how much is being redirected out of circulation due to stress (should be as low as possible)

- TPO and TgAb: thyroid antibodies (should be close to 0); elevations show potential auto-immunity to your own thyroid.

Blood Sugar Monitoring

If you are trying to lose weight, struggle with cravings, suffer from foggy thinking or lack of attention span, or wake up hungry, one of the simplest and most effective tests you can do is to track your blood sugar. Knowing how your body processes sugar, how quickly it uses it and stores it, and how your blood sugar reacts to specific foods (or food combinations) can be extremely helpful. You may quickly find that foods you thought were "healthy" for you are not. Conversely, foods you considered to be off-limits might work well for you.

Before you get started, you'll need some way to check your blood sugar. The simplest way is to get a blood glucose reader. These can be found at your local drugstore and do not require a prescription. You'll simply use a little pinprick on your finger to check your sugars. If, however, you are prediabetic or diabetic, you should ask your doctor to prescribe a continuous glucose monitor. This is a little device that you attach to the back of your arm. It will sync with your smart device and give you readouts throughout the day. You can even set your device to alert you if your blood sugar drops too low or spikes too high. There are more and more non-prescriptive continuous glucose monitors coming on the scene, so depending on what year you are reading this, you might just want to do a quick internet search for "purchase CGM."

Whether you are using a pinprick or a CGM, get started with checking your fasting blood sugar. Keep your device near your bed, and before you get up and rolling, take a measurement. This number, as I stated earlier, should be well under 100 mg/dL, and even closer to 80 mg/dL. Yes, it can get too low (under 70 mg/dL), but more often, we are concerned with this number being high.[21] That is because by the time you wake in the morning, your body should have long since

In a healthy metabolic state, you should wake up "ketogenic," which means mobilizing your booty and belly for energy, not getting your energy from sugar.

processed all sugar in your system and now be tapping into fat stores for energy. *In a healthy metabolic state, you should wake up "ketogenic," which means mobilizing your booty and belly for energy, not getting your energy from sugar.*

If you find that this number is higher than 90 mg/dL, start by paying attention to what you ate for dinner and when. Make sure that your prior meal was well balanced and early enough for you to have fully digested it before you went to bed. If that meal was too high in carbohydrates (for your personal chemistry), you might have ended up blowing through that sugar early in your sleep, then hitting a hypoglycemic level. If you pop up in the middle of the night suddenly, it's likely due to your blood sugar suddenly dropping, which signals your body to pump out the stress hormone cortisol. When cortisol elevates, it requires the body to start mobilizing sugar in order to handle the perceived stress. So even without eating sugar in the middle of the night, your body can mobilize sugar from its liver stores and flood the system again. *This cortisol/blood sugar relationship is also why you are starving all day when you suffer from a bad night's sleep.* In fact, just one night of miserable sleep can land your blood sugars in the prediabetic ranges the next day! Just one of the many, many reasons that sleep is so key to our health.

Once you get in the habit of taking your fasting blood sugar reading, you can start playing with how you react to your meals throughout the day. Before you eat a meal, check your blood sugar. This is your baseline, aka preprandial, reading. Make a note of this number, and make a note of all the components of your meal. After you eat, you'll want to take additional readings to see how your blood sugar reacts and how long it takes your blood sugar to get back to baseline. If your number spikes up (like 30 mg/dL) thirty minutes after your meal, it may have been way too high in sugar or starch for you.[22] And if your blood sugar stays elevated above your preprandial number for more than sixty minutes, I would suggest you completely rethink that food combo. You can take post-meal

> This coritsol/ blood sugar relationship is also why you are starving all day when you suffer from a bad night's sleep.

(postprandial) readings at 30, 60, 90, and 120 minutes, or until you see that baseline number return. This is where you can see that even things like "whole grain" or "high fiber" bread and cereals are not much better than their white and processed counterparts. Why? Because you may have the same level of blood sugar spike postprandial, but with white bread or sugary cereal, you may then drop back down pretty quickly. They give you a spike, but it's often short-lived. Plus, you are then craving more once your blood sugar drops. But with whole grain bread or muesli cereal, you may see that your blood sugar rises to a similar level but stays there longer. Sure, you may be full a bit longer, but that circulating blood sugar is wreaking havoc on your entire system by causing inflammation.

After you've spent some time working on getting your blood sugars under control and learning which foods work and which don't work for you, you'll be ready to take it to the next level. Remember, when you wake in the morning, having not eaten for ten or more hours, you should be approaching that "ketogenic state" I mentioned above. When your body is running on ketones (the by-product of breaking down fat for energy), you have a very efficient system. It is not a dangerous place to be; it is magical. Your brain is running on clean energy, and you may find that you have amazing clarity when you are ketogenic. You can play with how long you go from dinner the night before to breakfast the next day. As we discussed in the "Nourish" chapter, playing with a fasting window can reap wonderful benefits.

If you want to test your blood ketones, it can be fun to see how well you are tapping into your waistline for your energy needs. My favorite and most affordable (as of the writing of this in 2023) is the KetoMojo blood glucose and ketone monitor. It comes with strips for both readings so you can learn how your blood sugar and ketone readings correlate. I do not recommend you go straight to ketone monitoring from the get-go, as you need to get in tune with your blood sugar swings first. But if you are ready to really get down to the nitty-gritty after that, ketones will tell you a lot!

Heart Rate Variability (HRV)

Monitoring heart rate variability is a bit further out on the spectrum of self-quantifying. This refers to measuring the length of the space between heartbeats. If you are in a recovered, centered state (parasympathetic), you will have many variations in the length of time between your heartbeats. Contrary to what many, indeed I, believed, the heart should not beat like a metronome. The more static and unvaried the spaces, the more stressed, tired, and ill you are. Nowadays, you can get HRV data from high-end fitness trackers like Oura Ring, Garmin, or Whoop bands. When I first got into tracking this, you had to wear a special heart monitor with electrodes on your chest for three days. I used to work for a company based in Finland, FirstBeat, that was one of the first to develop HRV technology. I'd have clients wear the device for three days, send it off to the lab, and then I'd spend an hour sitting down with them to review the results. Now, you can just look at your app. Amazing!

If you are concerned that your current lifestyle is at the root of your ailments, or your doctor has been telling you to "watch your stress levels," this might be a good route to consider. Again, the question is, if you decide to track heart rate variability, what will you do with it? You better be willing to start a daily meditation or long walks with the dog when you see what your heart is dealing with all day. I can tell you right now I have never seen someone start tracking HRV and not be abashed by the data. Once you can see actual data points that show you how you're managing stress all day, it gets really hard to ignore. It's like, "Well, if I can't see the damage I'm doing to myself, then it might not be real."

But it is! And you should know about it. Being ignorant of our own ailments is not okay. So if you think that you might want to start looking at HRV, just go into it already knowing that you will need to make adjustments. You will be blown away, however, at how quickly you'll learn how to increase your HRV. You'll find that just getting to bed thirty minutes earlier, or skipping the afternoon coffee habit, are enough to give you a boost of a few points. *HRV is one of the easiest things you can improve wellness-wise, and it just so happens to be super important.*

It is even more helpful when used in combination with the other metrics mentioned above. If you are tracking blood sugar, you will be able to see how certain meals or foods not only spike your blood sugar but tank your HRV too. Sleep is key for keeping you out of "fight-or-flight" mode and more in "chill and relax" mode. You know how everything, even the tiny inconsequential things, are just so much harder when you are underslept? Your brain and body are just "hanging on" when you are that tired. That messes up your blood sugar big-time and leaves your stress hormones all out of whack, and you can bet your HRV is abysmal. This is an excellent example of how combining metrics can give you a full picture of all the things you can do to improve your wellness. On a day like that, you'd try to keep caffeine minimal, eat based on your "nourish" plan, get some light activity out in the midday light, and shut off all your screens to get your butt to bed early.

HRV is one of the easiest things you can improve wellness-wise, and it just so happens to be super important.

DNA Testing

Over the last decade or so, using your DNA to figure out what your health profile looks like has been picking up speed. From 23andMe to hundreds of software analytic websites,

Please understand that this data only tells you what your genes *could* be doing.

there is no end to the information they can tell you. DNA is being used to help people learn what foods they should choose, what exercise and sports they are best designed to do, and even what diseases they may be likely to get. It can be exciting and scary and all things in between. ***However, please understand that this data only tells you what your genes* could *be doing.*** There are genetics, and then there are "epigenetics." Your genes have proteins that can be activated and deactivated. What that means is that the things you eat, the air you breathe, and the movements you make can all affect whether some of these genes are turned on or stay turned off.

Obviously, there are genes that are just turned on and stay on. If you were born with big feet, you have big feet for the rest of your life. However, if you have the genes to eventually develop dementia, it doesn't mean you will suffer from it for sure. There are some choices that you make throughout life that will either cause those genes to get activated or stay dormant. The science of genetic testing and genetic expression is still developing. While we don't know exactly what you can do (or not do) to control how your genes are expressed, there is actually a fair amount of information we already know that can be helpful in making some basic decisions about your personal nutrition and exercise choices.

The science of nutrigenomics is about figuring out how your genes will likely respond to your nutrition. Will drinking wine lead you to develop breast cancer? Will having a high-fat diet cause obesity for you? Will eating a high-carb diet cause diabetes? Depending on your genetic profile, your answers to the above may be very different from mine. The data you garner from your genetic profile can also tell you how well you absorb B vitamins, metabolize fat and sugar, lay down good muscle tone, run fast, and even how old you're likely to live to. Recently, I got involved with a company called LifeDNA. They use your unique genetics to help you figure out what to eat, how to move, and what to expect longevity-wise if you do all you can to optimize your health.

The information can be fascinating! However, like all the other testing we discuss in this section, knowing *what* you will do with the information is even more important than getting the info. Be honest with yourself before you dig into gathering this information. Do you really want to know if you have a high likelihood of developing osteoporosis or diabetes? If you do want to know, will you be willing to make changes to help prevent these diseases? Honestly, I was not surprised by anything I learned once I got my profile done. It was mostly stuff I knew, and some of it was a good reminder that I needed to focus on certain nutrients and lifestyle choices. So, just take it all with a grain of salt.

Food Sensitivities

This is the testing I get asked about most frequently. We all know that there are foods we don't do great with, get digestive issues after eating, or even have all-out allergies to.

Keep in mind that being overly reactive to foods is a sympton, not a cause of your health issues.

Sensitivities to certain foods can be very disruptive, and figuring out your own nutritional triggers can really help alleviate a lot of health issues. I will go into detail below on how to use various food sensitivity testing. *However, keep in mind that being overly reactive to foods is a symptom, not a cause of your health issues.* We develop food allergies and aversions often because of underlying gut dysfunction, leaky gut, and even some other disease states. If you find that you are highly reactive to particular foods, please use it as a sign that it's time to talk to a functional health practitioner and start figuring out *why*.

Elimination Diets: These are where a lot of people get started. By eliminating a particular group of foods *for at least ninety days*, you can get an understanding of how your physiology is affected by it. After a complete avoidance of that food or food group for three months, you would then very strategically and scientifically reintroduce it back into your diet. For example, let's say you were concerned that dairy was something that was causing sinus, skin, and/or digestive issues. First of all, you'd take time to go through your fridge and foods you consume regularly and find things that will need to somehow be substituted with a non-dairy alternative. Then you'd need to get going on some new recipes and shopping lists. At first, it may seem almost impossible, but like most elimination diets, after a couple of weeks, you generally figure out some good options.

The real magic in elimination diets is twofold: (1) making sure to completely abstain from exposure for ninety days and (2) reintroducing it with a plan. Yes, some guides will recommend thirty days of abstinence, but I have found that it can take much longer for the gut to heal from years of exposure to something that has been causing inflammation. Giving yourself a good three months to both get

The real magic in elimination diets is twofold: (1) making sure to completely abstain from exposure for ninety days and (2) reintroducing it with a plan.

some new foods into the mix, and to allow the inflammation to heal, allows you to really see if, indeed, dairy (or
whatever you choose to experiment with) is causing your
symptoms. After that, having a solid plan for how and
when you'll reintroduce a food into your diet will help you
figure out if, for example, all dairy is off the table or just
certain types.

If I have a client eliminating dairy, then I would put
together a reintroduction chart for them. We would start
with the versions of dairy least likely to be problematic; test
small doses for three days or so, then go on to the next. So,
I'd have the client indulge in a tablespoon of clarified butter
three days in a row. They'd make notes on how they felt and
any symptoms or issues. If all was good, then we might go
on to butter for three days. Then either heavy cream or hard,
dry-aged cheeses. Then we would go to cultured yogurt or
kefir. Soft cheeses might come in after that. Finally, we'd play
with whole milk. Just trying to reintroduce dairy alone could
take a month! And that's if we didn't take goat and sheep milk
off the table.

The tediousness of eliminating for so long and then
reintroducing so slowly is the main reason I don't do a lot
of elimination diets with my clients. It can be a slow slog
and takes a lot of patience. In addition, it really requires the
participant to be actively paying attention to their symptom-
atology. If they don't notice that they have foggy thinking or
eczema coming back, then the reintroduction is just going

to be a waste of time. Instead, we often opt for doing some blood testing to see how the immune system is reacting to certain foods and food groups.

Blood Work: There are so many food sensitivity tests out there that you can order. You can even order many of them yourself. However, when I order testing for my clients, I try to ensure that we are gathering the right information and that the results will be actionable. Depending on one's symptoms, there are two different tests I like to order, and both tests require a blood draw. One is more general, and the other is quite granular. While at the moment these are my two go-to options, I'm always on the hunt for new ones.

Oxford Biomedical Technologies' Mediator Release Test (MRT): This test looks at your immune system's reactivity to 176 different food antigens (an antigen is anything that can cause an immune response). Essentially, they take a drop of your blood and measure the total volume of white blood cells in the sample. Then they let the sample react with one specific food antigen. Once the reaction is done, they remeasure the volume of your white blood cells. The greater the change, the more reactive you are to that particular food. Test results come back showing your reactivity using a bar scale, as you can see in the vegetable category example on the next page. Once we review these results, I then work with my clients to remove all the highly reactive and moderately reactive food antigens from their diets for ninety days. Then we either reintroduce as I discussed above or we retest the MRT.

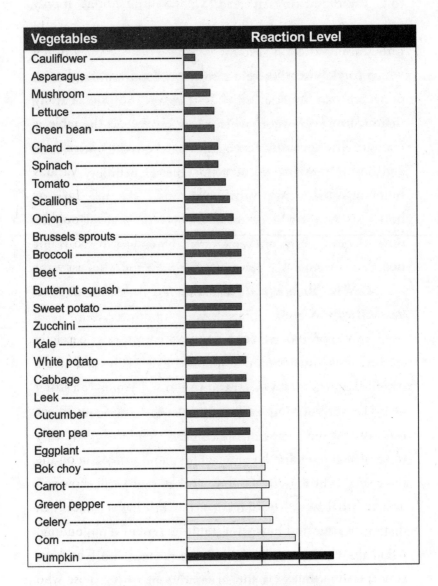

Sample from anonymous client's results in 2021

There are two drawbacks to this test. First of all, it only tells you about the whole food. For example, you would only learn if wheat is reactive for you. There's no way to tell which part of the wheat proteins (globulin, albumin, gliadin, or gluten) are the real culprit. For many, this doesn't really matter; just knowing that wheat should be off the table is enough. The second drawback is that you don't learn how your immune system is reacting to it, just that it is. Various immunoglobulins may be at work (IgA, IgD, IgE, IgG, or IgM). Knowing what type of immune reaction you should be wary of can be helpful to some, but for others, it too is not necessary. In general, I order an MRT for those who just want a good list of things to eliminate while we work on some good gut-healing protocols.

Vibrant Wellness' Food Zoomers: These tests do exactly what their name says: they "zoom" in on each food at the peptide level. I like to describe it like this: If you have a string of pearls around your neck representing a food you might react to, this test looks at each and every pearl individually to see which ones are the biggest issue. By zooming in on the individual peptides, the Zoomer profile results will show you not just what foods you're reacting to but what specifically in them is of issue and how your immune system is responding. I find these panels to be really helpful for clients who have very specific symptoms and/or conditions or for those who have already tried other elimination diets and tests before. In fact, I ran this test on myself (having already done the

MRT years before) and found that my go-to replacements for gluten (almond and corn) were becoming a serious issue for my immune system. My body was really burdened with inflammation from my overconsumption of what I thought were "safe" foods for me!

Food Summary						Blank Cell - Low Reactivity	● High Reactivity ● Moderate Reactivity Not Ordered or N/A						
	Food Name	IgA	IgG	IgE	IgG4	C3D	Peptide level sensitivity	Food Name	IgA	IgG	IgE	IgG4	C3D	Peptide level sensitivity
High Reactivity Foods ●	Corn	-	-	-	-	-		Dairy	-	-	-	-	-	
	Wheat	-	-	-	-	-								
Moderate Reactivity Foods ●	Almond	-	-	-	-	-		Intestinal Perm.	-	-	-	-	-	
	Macadamia nut	-	-	-	-	-		Pistachio	-	-	-	-	-	
	Walnut	-	-	-	-	-								

Overview page from my Zoomer results in 2021.
While I do not have specific "allergies" to these foods, I am showing "peptide-level" sensitivity to each. Note, this is a seventy-four-page report, which then breaks down each food category into single peptides.

Metabolic Typing: One simple but effective way to figure out generally what types of foods and food combinations work best for you is to take the Metabolic Typing Test. This is a simple questionnaire that uses body type, blood type, heritage, fat deposition, and so on to help you dial in the best type of diet for you. While this doesn't really address food sensitivities or allergies per se, it does often explain why, for example, you didn't lose any weight on a keto diet while your spouse lost thirty pounds! I find that using this in conjunction with the aforementioned testing is a great way to really fine-tune diet recommendations for my clients. If you are interested in learning more about this, go to MTDiet.com.

Hormone Balance or Dysregulation: This is a big one. So big that I'm not really sure where to start. When I say hormone testing, I don't just mean estrogen and testosterone. We have stress hormones, thyroid hormones, hunger and satiety hormones, and on and on. Hormones are chemical messengers. They take information (signals) from your brain and send them to the responsible gland to execute the command. While hormone testing is not a new concept, how to test it is evolving. It used to be that doctors would just rely on blood samples to tell your hormone levels. However, we have learned that this can be problematic, especially with stress and sex hormones. Taking a single blood sample on a random day and time give you only a snapshot, a quick peek at what your hormones are doing at the moment. It tells you nothing about the rest of the day, the week, the month, or even how they are being used throughout the body.

I like to see what is happening in the big picture: Is your brain sending signals to make the hormones? Is the particular gland able to produce said hormones? If so, how much? Can those hormones be used well by your body's cells? And most importantly, is your body then able to

detoxify those hormones? On top of all this, many practitioners don't take into account that all your hormones
are intricately interconnected. If your thyroid hormones
aren't optimal, your sex hormones will also suffer, as will
your stress hormones. If your stress hormones are out of
whack, the same will go for your sex and thyroid hormones.
This all sounds really oblique, I know, but I'll go into some
detail below to help demystify hormone testing and why
you should consider it.

Thyroid Hormones: Your thyroid gland production
is responsible for your basal metabolic rate. Without sufficient thyroid hormone production, you would not be able
to survive. In fact, if someone has their thyroid hormone
removed, they must be on replacement hormones for the
rest of their life! For those of us with a thyroid gland, the
body usually does a pretty good job of knowing how much
of the hormone to produce and when. Here is a basic expla-
nation of what happens in the body to get the thyroid functioning well:

1. TSH (thyroid-stimulating hormone): The pitu-
   itary gland signals to the thyroid gland to start
   making some thyroid hormone. This signal should
   be rather quiet. Your thyroid gland should hear
   the signal easily and produce enough hormones in
   response. If the signal is getting louder (i.e., your
   test result is higher), then we have a problem either
   with the signal being heard by the thyroid gland

or in its ability to make more thyroid hormone.[23]

2. Production of thyroid hormones (T3 and T4): The thyroid gland then produces mostly thyroxine (T4) and some triiodothyronine (T3). T3 is the most active form of thyroid hormone, and T4 will need to be converted in the liver, gut, and other tissues into T3. Some of these T4 and T3 hormones will be bound up or even used up by other functions in the body. Stress, in particular, can cause T3 to be sort of stolen (this is referred to as Reverse T3).[24]

3. Autoimmunity to thyroid: For many, there can be an issue with how well the thyroid gland is functioning due to autoimmune reactivity. This can be measured by looking at two different antibodies: thyroid peroxidase antibodies (TPO) and thyroglobulin antibodies (TgAb).[25] Autoimmune issues comprise a large percentage of why most people end up on thyroid hormone replacement.[26]

As you can see, there is a lot going on to get enough thyroid hormones made, converted, and then utilized by the cells appropriately. Sadly, when you go to the doctor to get your thyroid checked, they often look only at TSH. This makes me so frustrated! I can't tell you how many people I have met with who have underlying thyroid issues and

As you can see, there is a lot going on to get enough thyroid hormones made, converted, and then utilized by the cells appropri-ately.

autoimmunity who would have never known if they didn't insist their doctor order the other tests. Quite often the symptoms of hypo-thyroidism (sluggish thyroid) are very similar to those of depression:

Fatigue
Foggy thinking
Lack of libido
Dry skin
Weight loss resistance
Cold hands and feet
Hair loss
Weak or brittle nails
High cholesterol
Constipation

I speak from experience on this one. My mother's hypothyroidism was left undiagnosed for many years, simply because she didn't "look" like she had a meta-bolic issue. As hypothyroidism is often a genetic trait, it turned out I, too, would struggle with it. However, even though my TSH was high-ish at 4.8, doctors refused to medicate me because I was thin. Only when I found a functional health-minded doctor, who was concerned that

my inability to conceive a child was related to my hypothyroidism, was I finally put on medication. Had I not
found him (thank you, Dr. Richard Lee), I wouldn't have
my beautiful daughter!

If you are concerned at all that you need a closer look
at your thyroid function, below is a complete list of items
to request from your doctor, along with optimal lab ranges
for each. Note: the ranges I list below are taken from a
course I took in Functional Diagnostic Nutrition. These
lab ranges are based on functional/optimal health ranges
and will likely differ from those of your doctor's office:

- TSH: 1.4–2.2 mU/mL
- Total T4: 6.0–12.0 mcg/dL
- Free T4: 1.4–18 ng/dL
  (ideally in the upper half of this range)
- Total T3: 100–180 ng/dL
- Free T3: 3.4–4.4 pg/mL
  (ideally in the upper third of this range)
- Reverse T3: <15 ng/dL (as close to 0 as possible)
- TPO: <10 IU/mL (or as close to 0 as possible)
- TgAb: <20 IU/mL (as close to 0 as possible)

If you cannot get your doctor to order these, please
find a practitioner who will. Again, you can search for
someone at FDN Thrive or the Institute for Functional
Medicine.

Please know that just because you may have thyroid numbers that are out of balance doesn't necessarily mean that you will end up on thyroid replacement therapy. Without a prescription, there is much you can do with a functional health practitioner to get your thyroid working better. This would include working on gut and liver health, optimizing your mineral and nutrient density through diet and supplements, and quelling inflammation.

Your body and metabolic needs are in constant flux.

If you are already on thyroid replacement, you need to make sure that you are getting labs redone at least twice per year. *Your body and metabolic needs are in constant flux.* Stress, lifestyle changes, diet, exercise, and other hormones all affect how your thyroid is functioning and vice versa. Do not accept a simple TSH check either. Ask your doctor to run a full panel *every* time you get your thyroid checked. Otherwise, you won't know how your current prescription is working for you. Lastly, make sure not to let them only treat you based on your lab results. *The lab results must correlate with how you feel.*

The lab results must correlate with how you feel.

Sex Hormones: Your sex hormones play a role in much of your vitality, regardless of age. When thinking about sex hormones, estrogen and testosterone are probably the two hormones that pop into your head first. However, they are really only part of a very large and complex picture. A good practitioner will also want to know about your progesterone, DHEA, melatonin, and cortisol (just to name a few). They will want to see not only how much of these hormones you are making but, most importantly, what your body is doing with them!

As I discussed above, your body not only produces hormones but also has to use them and eventually excrete them. My favorite test for looking under the hood on this stuff is the DUTCH (Dried Urine Test for Comprehensive Hormones). This test helps me see so much. I have yet to run it on anyone and not have actionable information come from it. Not once! For example, I can tell if a woman is "estrogen dominant" because she doesn't have enough progesterone to balance her out. I can tell if a man is aromatizing (meaning converting) his testosterone to estrogen. I can see if clients aren't making enough melatonin to get a good night's sleep. I can even see if they are having a hard time detoxifying their estrogens and may need some support to avoid an increased risk of certain cancers! Below I include two pages from a DUTCH result that I got a few years ago. This one is from early on in my quest to feel more vital and regain some bone density.

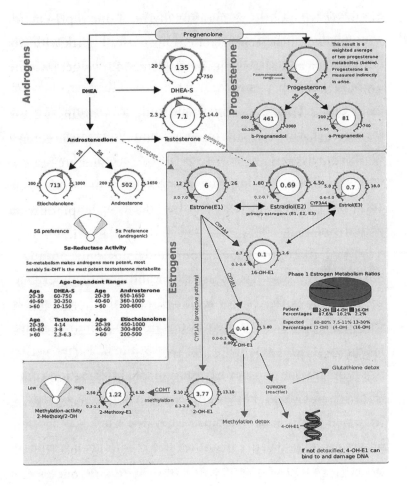

While I don't expect you'll be able to garner much insight from looking at those dials, I sure can. I know which ones should be balanced. I know where there are kinks in the chain. However, even the untrained eye can see that this gives you *way* more information than you might glean from a simple blood test. I continue to retest myself every six to twelve months to monitor my hormone replacement, supplements, diet, and exercise. Of course, I work with my own doctor and always put the information we get into the context of *me!*

Stress Hormones: Basically, this just means we are looking at what your adrenal glands are doing. Your adrenal glands are located at the top of each kidney and are responsible for so, so much! Not only do they pump out stress hormones, but in late life they also take over the production of sex hormones. These little powerhouses are critical to your longevity, vitality, and energy.

You can test these stress hormones with the DUTCH as well. You may have had your stress hormones checked by a doctor in the past using an Adrenal Stress Index or similar saliva test. The reason I, again, prefer the DUTCH here is it not only tells me the cortisol (your main stress hormone) but also the cortisone levels. Cortisone is the inactive form of cortisol. The body actually uses an enzyme to deactivate cortisol sometimes. In fact, if you have been overloaded with stress for a long time, you might start to inactivate your cortisol production preferentially. Why? Because having a high level of cortisol for too long can lead to devastating health outcomes. This is something I often see with my chronic exercisers who aren't balancing their recovery with their workouts.

I should step back here, though, and tell you that cortisol is not the enemy the media makes it out to be. We need cortisol to function. You need a fair amount of it to even get out of bed in the morning. You need it to get your butt in gear when things are gnarly. *We just need to make sure that you have a good pattern of cortisol through the day: a good hit of it in the morning, a waning dose throughout the afternoon, and little to none at night.* On a separate page of the DUTCH test, you can see what my cortisol and cortisone look like throughout the day.

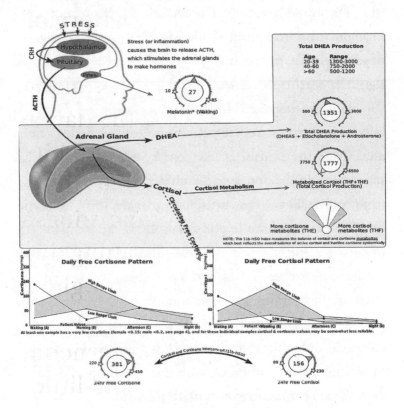

You can see how my "Daily Free Cortisol Pattern" line is almost flatlined in the graph on the right. I was chronically stressed, tired, and obviously hanging by a thread. If your line is flat, or worse, flipped (high at night), not only do we need to work on fixing that, but we really need to figure out *why!* Why is your cortisol rhythm suffering? And also, does this match how you feel?

We also look at your DHEA. Dehydroepiandrosterone is like a counterbalance to cortisol. If we think of cortisol as a breaking down (catabolic) hormone, DHEA is the building-up (anabolic) foil. If you don't have sufficient DHEA, you won't be able to keep any muscle tone, recover from colds, and so on. DHEA also feeds into the production of sex hormones like testosterone and estrogen. Looking at the chart on the previous page, you can see that my DHEA production was about the only thing I had to keep me going.

Having the larger context of how sex, stress, and thyroid hormones are all working together and how they affect one another is

We just need to make sure that you have a good pattern of cortisol through the day: a good hit of it in the morning, a waning dose throughout the afternoon, and little to none at night.

Having the larger context of how sex, stress, and thyroid hormones are all working together and how they affect one another is like doing a thousand-piece puzzle in a 3D matrix.

like doing a thousand-piece puzzle in a 3D matrix. Yes, it is complex, but boy, I love it. When I can look into that matrix and find details to illuminate why someone has been feeling "off" or not themselves, it's like winning the lottery for me! Suddenly those nagging symptoms and inexplicable ailments all fall into place. When I can finally illuminate for someone why they haven't been feeling so great and, more importantly, give them actionable steps to take to feel better, it is priceless!

Stool Testing

Many of you are familiar with the idea of stool testing. In fact, you may have had this done at your gastroenterologist's office. The real problem with some of the basic stool testing done in Western medicine is that it doesn't look very deep. A truly comprehensive stool test will not only look for a whole host of possible pathogens and even look for the proliferation of beneficial gut bugs but will also look for things like gut inflammation (calprotectin), immunity in the gut (secretory IgA), and enzyme sufficiency. *Ideally, you would get a complete picture of all the good, bad, and ugly going on in your gut.*

Diagnostic Solutions Laboratory GI-MAP (gastrointestinal microbial assay plus) is my preferred test. This test will give us a deep dive on parasites, bacteria, fungi, yeast, overall gut health, and immunity, and leave us with actionable changes to make. We'll be able to see which of those gut bugs are good and need to be cultivated. We will make a plan to eradicate the not-so-nice ones. We will figure out how to restore the integrity of the gut lining and thus enhance your immune system. When this test is done in conjunction with food sensitivity testing, we can get a very complete picture of how to make dietary changes to support your long-term health.

What we still don't know about the ideal ratios of healthy gut bugs is a lot. I'd like to comment on the current trend with many tests being advertised on TV. While I am quite excited that the general population is becoming more and more interested in the health of the gut biome, that doesn't mean we have an exact recommendation for each and every person. It's one thing to work with a practitioner to deal with nefarious critters in your gut and try to get some good healthy ones in there. However, we are still quite far from being able to tell you that you need specific ratios of each different biotic strain. If you've been interested in testing yourself using one of these services that analyze your gut microbiome, take the results with a grain of salt.

Organic Acids Testing (OAT)

This is a simple urine collection that can illuminate how your body's cells are functioning metabolically. Energy production, detoxification, neurotransmitter breakdown, and even activities of the intestinal microbes all have metabolic by-products. These are known as organic acids. When measured, they can tell you things like how you're digesting and assimilating your food, how efficiently your brain is working, how much energy you are producing, if you are having a hard time with environmental toxin exposures, and of course, how well your gut is functioning.

When I took this test myself, I was stunned at how much info I got. For example, I learned that I was getting quite a bit of mold exposure in the house we were renting at the time. It was old and dank, and I found that I had been struggling with chronic sinus issues ever since we moved in. This test was telling me that my cells were really struggling to clear this toxic exposure. Not only did I start taking some additional supplements to help with these specific detox pathways but I focused my efforts on really cleaning up the mold. What a difference it made!

Basically, anyone who is already working on eating well, managing stress, exercising the right amount, and still doesn't feel great should consider looking at what is happening at the cellular level. The OAT can help illuminate hidden healing opportunities for those dealing with

- Weight loss resistance
- Chemical sensitivities
- GI complaints
- Autoimmunity
- Low energy/metabolism
- Chronic fatigue
- Fibromyalgia
- ADD/ADHD
- Neurodegeneration
- Cognitive decline
- Autism
- Psychiatric disorders

Subtle abnormalities in metabolic health can be the result of enzyme, substrate, or cofactor deficiencies. Without getting too far into the weeds here, all cellular metabolism basically goes like this:

1. A substrate provides the raw material for a chemical reaction to occur.

2. Then, an enzyme causes the reaction to happen.

3. The enzyme uses a cofactor as fuel for the reaction.

4. Finally, there is a product from the reaction (and by-products).

If we see any enzyme that suggests dysfunction, we'll do the following:

- See what other enzymes in that category are doing. Meaning, if there's one aberration in all your gut function enzymes, and you have no symptoms, then it's less of a concern. But if you have a whole bunch of enzymes malfunctioning in the gut and you complain of symptoms, next we'll look at:

- What diet and lifestyle changes we can make to help you get the substrates and cofactors you need for that enzyme(s) to function better.

- We might look at your genetic profile (if you have one done) to see if you are predisposed to having issues with that particular enzyme's function.

Lastly, I might suggest temporary supplementation to help supply you with substrates and/or cofactors to help that enzyme function more efficiently.

All that mess means is that once we get you firing on all cylinders, you might feel better! You may find that you can clear up foggy thinking or your moods stabilize. Maybe some of your GI distress abates, and you lose a few pounds. I'm always blown away at how an organic acids test can illuminate areas that can affect your wellness in ways we may never have thought of.

Putting It into Action

With so many possibilities for testing, which should you consider (if any)? I realize it can be a lot to take in, not to mention the costs associated with each. My training at FDN ingrained in me the principle of "test, don't guess." I was also encouraged to run several tests at once with clients to maximize their results and actionable changes. This definitely can be helpful, but I have found over the years that it's best to start simple. I generally begin with comprehensive blood work for my clients. This will give us insights into possible infections, immune system struggles, thyroid and sex hormones, and even nutritional status. Then, depending on their symptoms, I might suggest additional testing.

For women, I almost always get a DUTCH test ordered to see what is going on with stress and sex hormones. This can be helpful for men as well, especially if they are struggling with excess weight and/or erectile dysfunction. For many, simply working on the principles in the "Nourish" chapter of this book will be enough to help them with diet struggles. But if there are severe and/or chronic digestive issues, a GI-Map is the next thing on our order list. Additional food sensitivity testing can often be helpful when coupled with a GI-Map to further eliminate troublesome foods. I order Organic Acids Testing less often these days, but not because it doesn't help; it's just not as easy to explain why someone might need it. But for those who've struggled, even after making changes to diet, rest, exercise, and stress management, OATs can often fill in the blanks on what might be missing.

> It costs a lot less to do some testing now than to pay to treat an illness later.

If you are committed to working with your practitioner on uncovering your own hidden healing opportunities and really owning your wellness, don't let the cost of running a few tests slow down your progress. Do it. Test, don't guess. Sit down and look at your results with your practitioner and really put them into the context of you! Make sure that you don't end up just treating the test results. Work on making changes that make sense for how you feel now and how you hope to feel in the future. ***It costs a lot less to do some testing now than to pay to treat an illness later.***

To help you figure out where you might want to focus your energy and laboratory budget, I have put together a chart below with each of the testing options we've discussed. Based on your current goals and symptoms, it might help you decide which one(s) may be a priority for you. Don't forget to consider not only your goals but *why* you want to reach them!

Test	What It Measures	Notes on Your Goals (and Why)
Basic Blood Panel	*Insights into immune function, nutritional status, detoxification, etc. A good starting point to decide on additional testing.*	
Blood Sugar Monitoring	*How your personal chemistry is reacting to the foods you are eating, how you're reacting to stress, and even how sleep affects metabolism.*	
DNA Testing	*How your genetics might be predisposing you to certain disease states, metabolic function, food sensitivities, etc.*	
Food Sensitivity	*Instead of labeling foods as "good" or "bad," find out how individual foods and food groups impact your personal health.*	
Hormones (Thyroid, Sex, Stress)	*How are these chemical messengers affecting one another, and how might they need balancing?*	
Stool	*Additional insights into gut function and integrity, and how it impacts your immune system and overall health.*	
Organic Acids	*Information on how your cells are working: Do they have enough raw materials, are their enzymes working, and what substrates are they producing?*	

CHAPTER FOUR

Enhance

Now, we get to chat about all the extra fun stuff: enhancements to your wellness journey. You may have noticed that I have yet to discuss any kind of supplements, and there's a good reason for that. If you aren't laying the groundwork by nourishing yourself well, moving your body, and dealing with nagging issues by exploring what's going on under the hood, there is no pill or potion in this world that will help you. You can't just pop supplements and sprinkle superfood powders on everything. Only after you have dialed in all the other things we've discussed so far should the extra enhancements come into play.

Just like every other section of this book, when it comes to enhancing your wellness journey, we need to do so keeping in mind your goals and your "why." I can't tell you how many clients have told me they honestly don't know why they are taking a pill. Maybe they had it recommended years ago by a doctor or a friend and they just kept taking it. There was one lady I went to visit at home years ago. We ended up doing a supplement audit of her fridge and cupboard. She was a very accomplished professional, now retired, and striving for optimal health her whole life. I have *never* seen a collection of pills and tinctures like that in my entire life. Between things that were expired, redundant, and some that were just downright unhelpful or borderline bad for her, we must have chucked at least $500 worth of wannabe health supplements. I was appalled and actually kind of sad for her. It's easy to buy into the hype. It's tempting to try a supplement that worked magically for your best friend. You can walk into any supplement aisle at Whole Foods and easily walk out with hundreds of dollars of promises and hopes.

Obviously vitamins, minerals, and all the other gobbledygook have some place in your health regimen. Once you feel like you are consistently eating according to your needs, moving well and often, and have figured out the root cause of some of your bigger health conundrums, it might be time to ask, What could I do to fill in some gaps? What is missing from my diet? What specific health needs do I have that cannot be managed solely with diet and exercise? *When you figure out what little extras you can put in to really maximize your health, supplements and other enhancements can really take your wellness to the next level.*

Know Why You Are Taking It

Why, why, why?! I know you are probably sick of my constant use of your "why," but I just can't help myself. It is so critical to your success in every aspect of your health. Right before I sat down to work on writing today, my husband was chastising our niece, "Don't ask why questions!" I laughed so hard. Sometimes he's right about that, but not when it comes to making very important decisions about your long-term health. When it comes to personal training, if I don't know why a particular exercise would benefit my client, I don't do it with them. Same goes for supplements. *If you don't know why you should take something, don't!*

> If you don't know why you should take something, don't!

I'll help you figure out a few options for yourself later on in this section. However, I will probably miss a few things that you have questions about. Please, please, please find yourself a health coach or functional/holistic practitioner to guide your decisions when it comes to your supplements. Not only can they help you find specific products for your unique needs but they can also help you find good quality options. I implore you not to buy your supplements from a drugstore shelf or third-party seller on Amazon. Yes, you may save a few dollars, but you have no guarantee about what you are actually getting. Not only might the product not contain what you think, but it might be formulated with fillers and stabilizers that aren't good for you at all. If you are going to purchase them on your own, look for those that are either CGMP (Current Good Manufacturing Practices) certified or have an independent third-party COA (Certificate of Analysis). A COA by NSF, BSCG, USP, or Consumer Lab will help ensure that you are getting something that (at the very least) contains what you think it does.

Don't just reorder.

Once you are taking something for a good reason and have found a quality product, I recommend you reevaluate your need for it after a while. One way to do this is just to let the product run out before you purchase a refill. That will give you a chance to take a week or so off and see how you do without it. Unless the supplement is doctor prescribed, it will probably be good to take a rest from it for a short bit. I usually order my supplements from an online dispensary and avoid the auto-renew option for exactly this reason. It's just nice to take a little break and make sure I even need it.

Look for redundancies and synergies.

Checking for duplication is a good way to thin out your medicine cabinet. I often see clients taking a multivitamin but also taking a few isolated supplements that are actually already in their multi. For example, if your doctor wants you to take a vitamin D supplement, but you already have the full dose they recommend in your multi, there's no need for both. Also, when we take a single vitamin or mineral all by itself, we often run the risk of causing new deficiencies. Sticking with our vitamin D example: You have likely heard that you need some magnesium to allow for proper vitamin D utilization. However, you also need sufficient vitamin K, calcium, and selenium. In nature, we don't ever get a single vitamin or mineral in a high dose. It always comes in a package with tons of other nutrients that all work together. When you isolate just one, then the body often has to pull the other synergistic nutrients from somewhere else (your blood or bones usually). *So just be careful with taking single nutrients; you may find that you'd be better off just reaching for whole foods instead.*

> So just be careful with taking single nutrients; you may find that you'd be better of just reaching for whole foods instead.

Watch out for interactions.

On the other side of this is that taking a certain vitamin can actually negatively interact with other medications. I know many women (myself included) who take thyroid medication in the morning. If we ingest calcium or iron within one hour of our meds, we will inhibit the absorption of the thyroid hormone that we need to function. Luckily, most doctors are good about telling patients about interactions like these. However, sometimes they are less obvious. Ask your pharmacist or prescribing doctor if there are supplements or even foods you should be wary of interacting with your medications.

Be strategic.

When starting a new supplement (or a bunch of them), it is really important to layer them in strategically. Remember, while they may be over-the-counter products, most of them are quite powerful. Don't just start taking five new things all at once at the highest dose recommended. If/when you have a negative reaction, you'll have no idea which of them or which combination of them is the culprit. To avoid this blind faith, start with a supplement protocol. I always devise a titration chart for my clients. I order the supplements based on the highest priority. Then I have them start with the minimal dose for three days. After that, we incrementally layer in the next higher dose of that one supplement until we have reached the maximal dose I originally recommended. Only after that would they start the process again with the next supplement in the chart.

If, for example, my client felt fine at half the recommended dose, but at the full dose noticed some nausea, we could then drop back to the half dose. Once symptoms subside, they could then stay at the lower dose and continue on to the next supplement. Sometimes people notice that they don't feel well when taking certain things. I'm often surprised to hear that a client had a really bad reaction to a supplement I normally regard as benign. But this is exactly the point. Each person is unique: our digestion, genetics, sensitivities, and so on are all factors in how our bodies process various chemicals. Again, this is another reason why vitamin X might have worked wonders for your buddy and did zippo for you.

Below is an example of a titration chart I recently gave to a client. The supplements were actually recommended by her general practitioner, but she felt overwhelmed. So I put this together for her to help her layer them all in. I ask my clients to print out their chart and post it near the vitamin cupboard. They can easily make notes on how they felt and the correct dosages for themselves.

Supplement Titration Chart

**Start with lowest dose, and increase slowly
every two to three days until maximal dosage.**
Do not go to next supplement without
completing titration of previous.

Supplement by Priority	Starting Dose	Maximal Dose	Timing/ Instructions	Reason for Taking	Notes
1. Vitamin D3	1/day after dinner		After meals	Increase blood levels, increase immunity and energy	
2. B12 Liquid	½ dropperful by mouth	1 whole dropper	In a.m. Try to hold in mouth about 30 sec. before swallowing.	Energy	
3. Berberine Complex	1 cap in a.m.	2 caps, 3x per day	On empty stomach, between meals	Healthy gut function, better blood sugar regulation	
4. DHEA	1 cap/day	2 caps/day	In a.m, or second one in midday	Support energy and balance cortisol production	
5. Micro Liposomal C	1 teaspoon in a.m.	1 teaspoon up to 3x/day	Empty stomach	Immune function, gut health	
6. Super K Elite	1 softgel after dinner		After dinner	Strong bones, good circulation	

As you can see, this sure cleans up the guesswork when it comes to figuring out how all these vitamins might be affecting you. I know this may look like a lot, but I've seen clients have even more supplements and tinctures recommended by their practitioners than this. Not only is it overwhelming to the client financially but trying to organize and remember when and how to take each is hard. This makes it simple and methodical. You can even use something like this for supplements you are already on. It's a good way to lay it all out for yourself, find redundancies, and remind yourself why you take that stuff to begin with. In the final chapter of this book, I have provided you with a titration chart to use. As an added bonus, when your doctor asks you what supplements you take, you'll already have a record of each.

Understanding What to Take (and Why)

In a perfect world, we would each take very specific supplement support carefully selected for our individual unique needs. However, I know that many of us will end up just buying a few things to take every day as "nutritional insurance." Regardless of what your friends tell you, or what commercials appeal to you on TV, there is actually some value in taking a few basics. Before you go online and start purchasing a multivitamin, I'd like to help you understand some general principles. Below I will outline for you simple information on what different types of supplements to consider, how they are best absorbed, and, of course, why you might consider taking them. At the end of this section, I will help you plug in which supplementation might fit best with your personal goals and *why's*. This is, by no means, a complete list of all the nutrient support you might consider, so, once again, please consult with your health practitioner

> Even if you take a wonderfully high-quality pill that is likely to boost your health, but you take it at the wrong time of day or with the wrong food, it's not going to help you.

before you purchase and start taking any of the below.

Note that once you figure out what supplements you should be taking and why they may be good for you, you still need to know how and when to take those magical pills. *Even if you take a wonderfully high-quality pill that is likely to boost your health, but you take it at the wrong time of day or with the wrong food, it's not going to help you.* It may even harm you. Many years ago, I remember a client telling me that he had been taking his doctor-prescribed fish oil every day and just hated the stuff. Every time he took it, he ended up with fishy burps and then couldn't drink his coffee. I had to stifle the giggles as I asked him, "Are you taking it first thing in the morning?" "Yes" was the reply. "Do you put anything in your coffee? Cream or similar?" "No," he said. Poor guy had been taking a fat-soluble supplement with no fat. There was no way he was going to be able to digest and assimilate all those omega-3s without some good fat to go down with it. While his doc had every good intention of helping him boost his antioxidants and gut health, he should have instructed his patient to take the pills with a meal.

To prevent you from ending up with issues like fishy burps, let me give you a few guidelines. I will go into some detail about certain vitamins, minerals, and other options. Please don't get bogged down in the science of each. At the end of this section, you will find a helpful chart with each supplement, what it does (i.e., why you should take it), notes on how to take it and what to combine it with (or not), as well as a place to make notes for yourself on those you want to consider. I will not get too detailed with the doses below. Please look at the labels for the "recommended daily intake" or RDI, or ask your health practitioner for advice on the correct dosage for your needs.

Water-Soluble Vitamins

Water-soluble vitamins refer to those your body cannot store for later use. They are easily absorbed into the bloodstream, and any that you don't use are usually peed right out. They have a relatively short-lived time to act: from a few hours up to a few days. Since you can't store them for very long, they'll need to be replenished regularly.[27] The water-soluble vitamins include vitamin C and all the B vitamins. These do not need to be taken with a meal (unless combined into a formulation with fat-soluble vitamins). Some of my clients report that they feel nauseous if they don't have food with these vitamins; please do what feels best for you.

Vitamin C

Also known as ascorbic acid, vitamin C is crucial to the immune system, connective tissue, and bone health, and works to fight free radicals as an antioxidant. Since our bodies cannot make any vitamin C, we have to take it in from food or supplements. Obviously you can get vitamin C from citrus fruits, but there's also plenty of it in cruciferous veggies. If you are a smoker, have a compromised immune system, or aren't very good at eating your veggies, you might consider taking more vitamin C. If supplementing, be aware that too much can cause GI distress. Aim for 1–3 grams per day.[28]

B-Vitamins

There are actually eight B vitamins that we need for optimal health, although vitamins B-6 and B-12 seem to get more of the spotlight. As a group, the B-Complex is needed for metabolic health, detoxification, transporting oxygen, and so much more. Without B vitamins, energy suffers, blood circulation slows, brain fog sets in, and a whole host of other issues come into play. If you are eating according to the principles we discussed in "Nourish," you are likely getting plenty of all the B vitamins you need, especially if you are focused on nutrient-dense proteins. There is a high concentration of B vitamins in animal proteins, especially non-muscle meats (like liver, kidney, etc.) as well as fatty fish. Vegans and vegetarians, and anyone who has diminished digestive function (meaning they don't break down protein well) should consider taking a B-complex. Women who are looking to get pregnant, are pregnant, or are breastfeeding should also take methylated folate (5-MTHF) to help with healthy fetal development.[29]

Some people are genetically predisposed not to absorb and utilize some of these B vitamins very well. If you have ever done a genetic test (as we discussed in "Explore"), you might already know if you have the MTHFR mutation. If that is the case, you will want to supplement only with B vitamins that are in their methylated form. (The MTHFR mutation means you are lacking a critical enzyme to utilize these vitamins).[30] They are a bit more expensive, but taking the synthetic versions of these B vitamins will not benefit you at all. I actually do not have any issues with methylation genetically; however, I take only methylated forms of B vitamins because they are so highly absorbable, and I know that I'll get out of them what I paid for. You'll occasionally hear doctors recommend you take one of the below B vitamins for specific deficiency issues. However, if you are looking to just ensure you are getting an adequate intake of each, look for a complete B-complex that contains all eight.

Here are the eight B vitamins and a note about what they do, as well as the best food sources for each:[31]

- Thiamin (B1): Essential for helping derive energy from your food. Abundant in pork, sunflower seeds, and wheat germ.

- Riboflavin (B2): It also aids in making energy from the food you eat as well as having antioxidant powers. Find it in organ meats, beef, and mushrooms. The active form of this is *riboflavin-5-phosphate*.

- Niacin (B3): Plays a role in how cells communicate with one another, energy production, and creating and repairing DNA. Found in chicken, tuna, and lentils. You may see it as *niacinamide*.

- Pantothenic Acid (B5): Like the other B vitamins, we need this to help release energy from our food. It also helps with making hormones from cholesterol. It's found in liver, fish, yogurt, and avocado. Find the absorbable form as *calcium d-pantothenate*.

- Pyridoxine (B6): We specifically need B6 to break down proteins into amino acids. Those amino acids are used to make neurotransmitters (brain signaling) that are also assisted by pyridoxine. It aids in the creation of red blood cells as well. Chickpeas/garbanzos, salmon, and potatoes are all high in B6. Supplements should be in the form of *pyridoxal-5-phosphate* or *pyridoxine-HCl*.

- Biotin (B7): Critical to carbohydrate and fat break-down. It also affects gene expression (how your DNA shows up in real life). You can get B7 from yogurt, cheese, eggs, salmon, and liver.

- Folate (B9): This B vitamin is critical to many health functions: breakdown of proteins (amino acids), creation of both red and white blood cells, and of course, cell growth and development, which is why it is important for expectant mothers. Liver, leafy greens, and beans are all good sources. Note that folic acid is a synthetic form of folate and less bioavailable. Look for 5-*methyltetrahydrofolate* instead.

- Cobalamin (B12): Your brain can't function well without enough B12. We also need it for DNA production and the creation of red blood cells. You can get it in meat, eggs, seafood, and dairy. Vegans and those who do not digest protein well are often deficient in cobalamin. Look for supplements in the form of *methylcobalamin*.

Fat-Soluble Vitamins

The fat-soluble vitamins include A, D, E, and K. These vita-mins can be absorbed only when consumed with fats, and preferably a little protein. These, however, can be stored in your body's liver and fat tissue for later use. For that reason, you do want to be careful how much you are taking, as it is possible to overdose. If you have had the misfortune of having your gallbladder removed, you are at a disadvantage in getting these vitamins from your food/supplements into your bloodstream, as we need bile to help digest them. Note: I would definitely put fish oils and omega fats into this category.

Vitamin A

We need vitamin A (aka retinol) for good vision, a strong immune system, proper cell growth, reproduction, and healthy mucosal membranes.[32] It is also a powerful antioxidant. You'll often find retinoids in skin care treatments for anti-aging and acne. This is another one that you'll need to supplement with if following a vegan/vegetarian lifestyle, as it is found only in substantial doses in animal foods like liver, butter, milk, and egg yolks. You may be familiar with a similar substance to retinoids called carotenoids. These can be converted into vitamin A in the body. You can get carotenoids from green leafy vegetables, some root vegetables (like carrots), and other yellow and orange produce. However, only about 10 percent of carotenoids can be converted into vitamin A.[33] So if you are going to try to get your daily dose, it's best to eat those colorful veggies in an omelet cooked in butter. Oh, that sounds amazing right now! Supplement with caution, as most people will be able to get enough from diet alone. If it is in a multinutrient supplement, make sure it is balanced with the other fat-soluble vitamins D, E, and K.

Lastly, if you are using any kind of retinol creams for your skin, you might want to hold back on supplementing with pills. You will absorb quite a bit through the skin and may risk toxicity.

Vitamin D

I'm not sure there could be a supplement more well-known or even more controversial than vitamin D. We all know we need it; we all hear our doctors tell us to take it and get our levels up. But why? And how? Well, we need vitamin D for almost every cellular function in the body. Not only does it help with the absorption of calcium and phosphorus for strong bones but it also helps with the immune system, keeps inflammation under control, and even aids in mood stabilizing.[34] The list of what it does is long, and deficiencies in vitamin D can be blamed in part for many, many ailments. But as we have begun to spend more time indoors, eat less of the foods that naturally have vitamin D, and have impaired gut function needed to convert sunlight to vitamin D, as a species we seem to be coming up short on this one!

First of all, you should know that vitamin D is technically a prohormone. That just means that it basically helps your body's hormones be expressed and function as they should. Without it, many of your body's cells would not have the basic inputs they need to function optimally. The main way we are designed to get vitamin D is from our skin's production of it from ultraviolet B rays. If your skin, like mine, is on the darker side or you avoid direct sunlight, you are already predisposed to not optimizing your intake. Others may have a hard time converting the sunlight into vitamin D due to an inability to digest fats well (again, vitamin D needs fat to be absorbed) or a lack of intake. The elderly and those who follow a low-fat diet should pay particular attention to their vitamin D levels for this reason. Ironically, obesity can actually impair your skin's ability to convert vitamin D, so those who are overweight are also likely to be deficient.[35]

Unless you have difficulty getting outside on your own, you should consider some direct sunlight in midday. I recommend my clients start with just five minutes of sun exposure on large parts of their body: torso, legs, and arms. Ramp up slowly to about fifteen minutes a day around noon. If this is not feasible for you, you might want to consider increasing your food sources of vitamin D. Best sources would be mushrooms, egg yolks, fatty fish, and liver.

Make sure that when you get regular blood work done that they are testing your vitamin D levels. Aim for a 25-hydroxy vitamin D3 level of 40–80.[36] I find that most people will benefit from getting their levels on the higher end of this range. Note, your doctor's lab report may state that anything over 20 or 25 is fine. Like the rest of the advice in this book, we are not aiming for "fine"; we want to live optimally! Also, please don't go crazy on supplementing with vitamin D alone. Remember, the fat-soluble vitamins all work together synergistically. I have recently read reports online of some people taking super-physiological doses of 40,000 IU or more daily! They end up with all kinds of health issues related to huge imbalances in calcium and phosphorus absorption: heart attacks, strokes, and even death! Look to take your vitamin D supplement along with all other minerals and fat-soluble vitamins with a meal, and preferably later in the day. Unless doctor prescribed, you will likely only need a basic intake in supplement form of about 500–1000 IU daily.

Vitamin E

There are several forms of the "tocopherols," or vitamin E. Of these, alpha-tocopherol is the best utilized by the body as an antioxidant. This form of vitamin E helps prevent cells from oxidative damage (premature aging) and keeps the immune system strong. Unlike vitamin D, you are far less likely to be deficient in vitamin E since it is so easily obtained from eating things like nuts, seeds, and some fruits and vegetables. However, if you are following a strict low-fat diet or are impaired in your ability to break down fats, you may need to look into upping your intake of alpha-tocopherol. Although, make sure to avoid doses over 1,000 mg, as it may cause excessive bleeding and interfere with blood-thinning medications like warfarin.[37]

Vitamin K (1 & 2)

If there was one vitamin that I wish more people knew about and supplemented with, it would be vitamin K. Specifically, vitamin K2 flies under the radar in its critical importance to our overall health. Some of you may be familiar with vitamin K1, which is known for helping with blood clotting. In fact, if someone is on a blood-thinning medication like Coumadin, they may be told to avoid dense sources of vitamin K1, which includes dark green, leafy vegetables. Deficiencies in vitamin K1 are relatively rare, and supplementing with it is usually not necessary.

Vitamin K2 functions very differently from its cousin K1. In fact, I wish there was a whole separate name for it, because often the people who need to supplement with it are told to avoid "vitamin K" due to its blood-thinning effects. While some animals (like cows) can readily convert K1 from plant foods into K2, humans are not very good at it. That doesn't mean we don't need it, though. K2 actually works more like a traffic cop for minerals like calcium. Without sufficient vitamin K2, calcium is not always properly deposited where we need it in bones and teeth but instead can end up in kidneys, arteries, or even amassing in joints. In addition to calcium metabolism, K2 helps with heart, skin, and brain health.[38] Foods high in vitamin K2 include natto (a fermented Japanese dish), cheese, eggs, butter, liver, beef, and chicken. With the exception of natto, none of these foods are vegetarian, so avoiding animal products would be a good reason to start supplementing with vitamin K2.

I started learning about vitamin K2 when I began my quest to get stronger bones. *I was appalled to learn how critical it was to my bone health, and yet not one single doctor or nutritionist had mentioned it to me.* Unfortunately, the medical community is locked into this idea that calcium intake is the only thing missing from one's ability to have strong bones. This is not only misguided but potentially dangerous. If you are concerned with bone health and start supplementing with calcium alone, not only will you not end up with stronger bones but you will likely end up with other mineral and vitamin deficiencies in conjunction with erroneously deposited calcium in your soft tissues.[39] On top of that, the food sources I noted above for vitamin K2 aren't always sufficient to cover your body's needs for it. Unless your dairy, beef, and chicken are all sourced from grass-fed/pastured animals, chances are that the animals weren't converting their own food into vitamin K2. That means your

I was appalled to learn how critical it was to my bone health, and yet not one single doctor or nutritionist had mentioned it to me.

protein will be deficient in it too. Other sources of vitamin K2 in the diet include sauerkraut, kimchi, kefir, and most other traditionally fermented products.[40]

In order to understand its uses better, I'd like to delve a little deeper into vitamin K2. There are actually two well-known subtypes: MK-7 and MK-4. While both forms are needed for proper calcium metabolism, they work a little differently in your body's tissues. In the bones, MK-7 produces hormones that aid in regulating bone growth and breakdown. MK-7 also gets used in the liver, aids in testosterone production, brain function, and exercise performance, and even keeps blood sugar in check. MK-7 is actually a precursor to MK-4. That just means that the body eventually turns MK-7 (and all other subtypes of vitamin K2) into MK-4. While MK-4 is really the master menaquinone at regulating calcium deposition, it appears that supplementing directly with it may not work so well. To cover my bases (since eating natto—ever—is not on the table for me), I take a supplement that includes both MK-4 and MK-7 in addition to K1. Note that certain medications like statins and blood thinners can impede your body's absorption and use of vitamin K.[41]

Minerals

Minerals differ from vitamins a bit. While vitamins (both fat-soluble and not) are broken down through cooking and/or digestion and assimilated into your system, minerals maintain their original chemical structure. Vitamins are organic; minerals are inorganic.[42] The major minerals include calcium, chloride, magnesium, potassium, phosphorus, sodium, and sulfur. Some of these minerals are best absorbed with some fat, others with protein, while some don't necessarily need to be coupled with anything. Calcium, for example, is best absorbed with fat (one of the many reasons I detest skim milk). Sodium, on the other hand, is easily absorbed without any food. *The main thing to remember about minerals is that taking too much of one can cause deficiencies in others.* Sodium in excess will be bound with calcium for excretion.[43] So if you're overdoing it with the salt shaker or processed food, your bones may suffer. This is why you'll often see mineral supplements in combinations that work synergistically.

Calcium

It's fitting to discuss this mineral first since we just concluded our chat about its much-needed accompaniment, vitamin K2. While we mostly think of calcium as being important for bones and teeth, we need it for so much more: muscle contraction (including the heart), nerve function, and blood clotting. The body needs to make sure there is a steady level of circulating calcium. This is regulated by your parathyroid hormone (PTH). Too little, and the body uses vitamin D to increase absorption of calcium in your intestines and tells the kidneys not to excrete so much out. If there's too much, PTH signals the opposite. Maintaining the right level of calcium can be impacted by some medications (like corticosteroids and chemotherapy), excess sodium in your diet, and even food additives like phosphoric acid in sodas.[44] If you have a hard time digesting fats in your diet or follow a low-fat diet, you may need to pay attention to how well you assimilate calcium as well as other minerals. This is also the case if you are taking acid reducers (like Prilosec) or have had your gall-bladder removed.

Most of us, even if we don't eat dairy products, should be able to get enough calcium from our diet. But remember, minerals aren't broken down and as easily absorbed as vitamins. The bioavailability of calcium (meaning how much your body can actually utilize) is only about 30 percent for even the best food sources. If your cup of almond milk says it has 300 mg of calcium, you'll likely get only about 90 mg at best. That said, the RDA for calcium listed on food labels does take this bioavailability issue into account. The other thing to consider is that some plant food sources of calcium may have a high level of "anti-nutrients" like oxalates and phytates. These can bind to calcium and prevent your ability to absorb it. The best way to deal with this is to just make sure you cook your dark green, leafy veggies and throw out the excess water. Sardines and other small bony fish are my favorite source of calcium since you are actually eating those tiny little bones. You can also get a good serving from chia seeds, edamame, tofu, soaked and sprouted almonds, cashews, other cooked legumes, and of course, dairy.[45]

If you have been told by your health practitioner that you need a calcium supplement, please, please, please pay attention. *Calcium, taken alone, can not only be unhelpful in keeping bones strong but can actually wreak havoc on your health.* It is critical that you take it with all the necessary cofactors for proper calcium metabolism and deposition in your body's soft tissues. Look for a multi-mineral and vitamin supplement that includes magnesium, vitamin D, vitamin K2, phosphorus, zinc, boron, potassium, vitamin C, and manganese.[46] At the time of writing this book, I am currently really into a product called Bone Restore with Vitamin K2 by Life

> Calcium, taken, alone, can not only be unhelpful in keeping bones strong but can actually wreak havoc on your health.

Extension. Regardless of the formulation you end up taking, remember to take it with a meal or right after. I prefer taking my bone restore formula after dinner.

Phosphorus

After learning how much calcium needs other minerals to work its magic, let me introduce you to phosphorus. This mineral works synergistically with calcium to ensure your bones and teeth are well mineralized. However, we also need phosphorus to aid our kidneys in proper excretion, to make and use energy in our cells, and to make the building blocks of DNA and RNA.[47] Luckily, most people can get a fair amount of phosphorus through diet alone. You can get your daily intake of phosphorus from most high-protein foods: meat, poultry, fish, dairy, eggs, and legumes.[48] It appears that phosphorus in animal protein is more bioavailable than that found in plants. Plant sources are generally high in phytic acid or phytates, which lower your digestive ability to absorb phosphorus.

Like all other fat-soluble vitamins and minerals, we have to be careful not to have an excess. When one mineral is too prevalent, it will throw off the balance of others. Nowadays, many food producers will use inorganic (meaning man-made) phosphates. Even though these synthetic forms are not as healthful as organic phosphorus, they are absorbed readily into our system. Avoid sodas, packaged foods, and fast foods with any additives named phosphoric acid, dicalcium phosphate, sodium phosphate, or any version of those. It's unlikely that one would have a deficiency in phosphorus unless they have an issue with a hyperactive parathyroid gland or have been starved for an extended period.[49]

Chloride

This mineral is needed to help our bodies regulate fluid balance. Most of us get plenty of it from salt in our food. Normally we should have our chloride levels balanced with potassium to prevent excess fluid retention or loss. Supplementation is rarely needed, except in instances of severe fluid loss, like diarrhea or heat exhaustion.[50]

Magnesium

This may surprise you, but magnesium is one of those very rare supplements I recommend to almost every single client! Due to depletion of magnesium in our soils, many of us are really deficient in it. We need magnesium for so many physiological functions: muscle and bone health, nerve function, mood, blood pressure, blood sugar regulation, energy production, and on and on. You can get magnesium from foods like nuts, seeds, legumes, dairy products, and green leafies.[51] If you suspect, however, that you aren't getting enough, you might notice symptoms like constipation, sleep disturbances, muscle weakness, fatigue, low mood, and even nausea. Depletion can also be caused by a poor whole foods diet, renal disease, use of antibiotics and chemotherapy, overactive parathyroid (which will also affect calcium levels), diabetes, and alcoholism.[52]

Finding the correct supplemental form of magnesium might be a bit tricky as there are different types to consider based on your needs. Here is a quick cheat sheet on the various forms and what each does:[53]

- Mg (bis) Glycinate: One of the most bioavailable forms. Increases sleep quality and does not have a laxative effect. A safe and effective option for deficiencies.

- Mg Citrate: Very popular and cheap; has a direct laxative effect, especially at higher doses.

- Mg Chloride: Works for detoxing cells and tissues; good to replenish magnesium stores. Oral versions can help with kidney function and increase metabolism. It can often be found in topical lotions and applied to sore muscles and cramps. I personally love Ancient Minerals' Topical Magnesium and use it on my sore feet and neck every night.

- Mg Carbonate: Also very absorbable; converts to Mg Chloride when digested by stomach acid. Great for those with GERD/indigestion as it has antacid properties.

- Mg Oxide: A cheaper but less well-absorbed version. It works well to combat constipation, but that's about it.

- Mg L-Threonate: May help with cognition and brain health. No digestive impact.

- Mg Malate: Easily digested and absorbed; good for those with fatigue, as it aids in energy production. It may have an impact on muscle relaxation.

- Mg Sulfate: Well-known in the form of Epsom salts. Good for muscle relaxation and constipation. Do not take it orally.

- Mg Orotate: A pricier version, best known for increasing athletic performance and output.

- Mg Taurate: Used for those with cardiovascular concerns; it is well absorbed and has no laxative effect.

- Mg Glutamate and Aspartate: Avoid these forms as they have some neurotoxic effects.

Potassium and Sodium

I put these two essential minerals together as they work in tandem. Together they help regulate fluid in our bodies. Sodium is responsible for the extracellular (outside the cell) fluid, and potassium is responsible for intracellular fluid (inside the cell). The correct balance of these two is needed for proper muscle contraction and blood pressure as well.[54]

In fact, more important than the absolute intake of potassium or sodium might be the balance of the two.

In fact, more important than the absolute intake of potassium or sodium might be the balance of the two. Most people are over-consuming sodium in the form of processed foods like bread (yes, a sneaky sodium bomb), preserved meats, and so on, while undercon-suming good sources of potassium (fresh fruits and veggies, seafood, and dairy).[55]

Before we go any further, keep in mind that salt and sodium are not the same! Sodium is just a mineral that is found in salt crystals. And the salt that food producers use is extremely high in sodium because it is cheaper and preserves their products longer. If you are using a quality coarse grain sea salt, ounce-for-ounce it will be lower in sodium than its processed counterpart. We need to have a little sodium in our diet and plenty of potassium to keep our fluid balance even. If sodium is too high, blood pressure will increase and the risk for heart disease and stroke will go way up.[56] If this is a concern for you, make sure that most of your sodium comes in the form of quality sea salt and that you are getting plenty of potassium in your diet. Reach for avocados, legumes, tomatoes, seafood, leafy greens, and skin-on potatoes.[57] These are all high-fiber and lower-carb options to ramp up your potassium intake. Yes, bananas have plenty, but the sugar hit might be a bit much for many of you. Rarely are sodium or potassium needed in supplement form, unless prescribed by your doctor.

Sulfur

I have saved the most unsuspecting fantastic mineral for last. When most of us think of sulfur, we probably almost feel like we can smell it in the air. Yuck! We are not talking about the hydrogen-sulfide gas stink you get from contaminated water; we are talking about a really important mineral for your health. I do apologize, though, because now you probably have the sulfur stink thing stuck in your head—oops. Sorry.

The mineral sulfur is crucial to our cells' ability to detoxify, build and repair DNA, and repair cellular damage. If you are eating a clean whole foods diet, you likely will get enough sulfur from allium vegetables (like garlic, onion, and leeks), cruciferous veggies (such as broccoli, asparagus, and kale), eggs, legumes, nuts and seeds, meat, seafood, and dairy. And having a diet high in

The mineral sulfur is crucial to our cells' ability to detoxify, build and repair DNA, and repair cellular damage.

sulfur-rich foods will help keep inflammation in check, keep your heart healthy, minimize muscle and joint pain, stave off some forms of cancer, and even reduce your risk of age-related cognitive decline.[58] How's that for a powerhouse mineral?

A Note about Electrolytes

You may have noticed that the above minerals are all electrolytes. These essential minerals help regulate your fluid balance (in and outside the cells) and are involved in many chemical reactions throughout your body. While some of you may think you need electrolytes only in extreme heat or exertion, we actually need them all the time to make sure we are well hydrated, yes, but also to keep almost every metabolic reaction our cells need to do running smoothly. Since our bodies are about 60 percent water, we probably ought to make sure we are paying attention to electrolyte balance. To help you keep the right electrolyte mix in your bodily fluids, your kidneys and sweat glands can excrete any excess.[59]

Have you ever wondered why you get muscle cramps when you sweat too much or are dehydrated? Well, that is because electrolytes, which hold both positive and negative charges, are essential to proper muscle contraction. Your body also uses electrolytes to help move fluid in and out of the cells, so if there is an imbalance, those chemical reactions won't work. You can actually overhydrate too and still throw these processes off kilter. If you drink water in excess of the rate that your kidneys and/or sweat can keep up with, you end up with similar issues.[60] This doesn't mean you need to run off and buy electrolyte enhancers for your water. Please do not spend money on that stuff! All you need is about one grain of quality coarse sea salt (not iodized salt) per 16 oz. of water. That's it. Don't add so much that you can taste salt. That sea salt has magnesium, sodium, potassium, and calcium all in perfect ratios to help you get that water into your cells without going straight through you. A splash of lemon or lime won't hurt either.[61] I do this all day long in my own water.

Trace Minerals

Many of you may be familiar with trace minerals. These include chromium, copper, fluoride, iodine, iron, manganese, molybdenum, selenium, and zinc. While microscopic compared to the major minerals, trace minerals are just as essential to your health. From keeping bones and teeth strong to carrying oxygen throughout your body to enhancing your immune system, trace minerals do all kinds of wonderful things for us. However, just like the major minerals, overdoing supplementation with one can cause deficiencies in others. So read your labels carefully and make sure that you aren't getting supernatural levels.[62] Most of these would not be supplemented individually unless you had a particular deficiency determined by your health practitioner. Instead, you'll likely see trace minerals added to multivitamin/mineral products altogether or in particular combinations. Below I will give you just a few tidbits on each.

Chromium

This trace mineral helps insulin work to keep your blood sugar in check. We also need it for proper carbohydrate and protein metabolism. You can get your daily dose by eating nuts, cheese, liver, veggies, meat, and poultry. Deficiencies and toxicities are not common.[63]

Copper

We need copper to keep bones and cartilage strong. It is also needed for our bodies to use iron effectively. If you're eating beef, organ meats, nuts, or beans, you are likely getting plenty. While most will say that copper toxicity is not something to worry about, I disagree! Having had a copper IUD implanted once, I literally had to fight with my doctor to get it removed because of the myriad of copper toxicity symptoms I was having. The brain fog, swelling, nausea, and headaches were nonstop. Some women are just more sensitive, and that was me. Just a word to the wise. "Natural" or not, listen to your body, folks! Go with your gut.[64]

Fluoride

I'm sure you already know about this one from your dentist.

We generally need some fluoride for healthy bones and teeth. In fact, many of you likely live in areas where your water supply is infused with it. I'm not sure I agree with this tactic. There is some evidence to show it can negatively impact thyroid function and parathyroid function when in higher doses.[65] I lean on the side of filtered water and fluoride-free toothpaste about half the time, but don't tell my dentist. (Sorry, Keith.)

Iodine

Without sufficient iodine, your thyroid gland will not work well. Since a healthy thyroid function is critical to metabolic, cognitive, and basically whole-body health, that means we really need iodine too. But don't rush out to supplement it. You can get enough through eggs, poultry, grains, dairy, and of course, sea vegetables. While I'm not a fan of iodized salt due to its taste and high sodium content, it has helped millions of people in developing countries to no longer suffer from iodine deficiency. However, most living in the United States and other developed countries are likely good on iodine. Unless you suffer from goiter, supplementing is not necessary.[66]

Iron

Of course, we know we need iron for strong muscles and to make our blood supply. However, iron deficiency is much more common than other trace mineral deficiencies. Without good iron levels, we will not thrive! If you have lost a good amount of blood (like a heavy menstrual cycle or childbirth) or follow a vegetarian diet, you might not have those levels up where you need them.[67] While you can get some iron from plant sources like dark green, leafy vegetables; nuts; and beans, it is far less absorbable.[68] The richest and most easily absorbed sources of iron are animal flesh; sorry, but that's just the way it is.

Manganese

Unlike iron, manganese is plentiful in plant foods. It aids in the metabolism of cholesterol, carbs, and protein. Manganese is needed for cartilage and bone formation and wound healing. We also require manganese to produce antioxidants that fight off cellular damage and free radicals.[69]

Molybdenum

This not-so-well-known trace mineral is actually quite necessary for the breakdown of amino acids (protein). In fact, deficiency in molybdenum is associated with gout. You likely are getting plenty, however, as it is in legumes, dairy, whole grains, poultry, meat, and fish.[70]

Selenium

This critical trace mineral is also a powerful antioxidant.

It helps protect our cells from damage via oxidation (like the browning of an apple). Selenium is crucial for thyroid hormone conversion (T4 into T3), immune function, and reproduction. A little-known benefit of selenium is that it can actually combat mercury toxicity.[71] That must be why nature was smart enough to put a healthy dose of it right there in your fish. You can also get selenium in other animal proteins like beef and poultry and some plant foods like nuts and seeds. In fact, Brazil nuts have one of the highest concentrations of selenium in any food.[72]

Zinc

I'm sure many of you have popped extra zinc when you are feeling under the weather. Aside from helping boost your immune system, we also need zinc for wound healing, bone metabolism, and fetal development. It's another useful mineral for the digestion and assimilation of protein, fats, and carbohydrates. A surprising benefit of taking zinc is that it has been shown to boost testosterone levels (even if you get enough in your diet).[73] Luckily for me, one of my favorite treats is the highest source of zinc: oysters. If those aren't your cup of tea, you can also get a good dose of zinc from shellfish, beef, pork, poultry, cashews, and chickpeas. One note—you might want to lay off the zinc when taking some antibiotics, as it can decrease their effectiveness.[74]

Antioxidants

I remember when people first started really taking supplements at home, and the word "antioxidant" was all the buzz. I've touched on this a bit already, as some of the vitamins and minerals already discussed are "antioxidants." That means they work against oxidation. Oxidation at a chemical level means that a molecule or atom is losing an electron. When an electron is lost, and there is an uneven number of them, we end up with a "free radical." Free radicals are unstable and highly reactive.[75] But you should know that this is a natural and normal consequence of reactions happening in our bodies all the time. Every time you digest food and turn it into energy, oxidation happens. Every time you exercise, there is also oxidation. Where we get in trouble, health-wise, is when we have an overabundance of free radicals (oxidative species) without a good balance of antioxidants. Things like chemical exposures in our environment, smoking, processed foods, alcohol, and radiation can all increase your free radicals. When free radicals are running amok, we end up with inflammation, cellular damage, and all manner of diseases.[76]

Suffice it to say, we don't want to end up with serious health issues just because we don't have enough antioxidants to combat the free radicals in our bodies. If you are nourishing yourself daily with colorful fruits and veggies, eating only healthy fats, and avoiding processed foods, you will likely not have to worry about taking additional antioxidant support. In fact, supplements may not work nearly as well as food when it comes to antioxidants.[77] As good as our science is, there may still be unknown cofactors and other chemicals in foods that allow our bodies to more efficiently use those antioxidants to combat inflammation. In fact, we already know that there are hundreds, maybe even thousands of chemicals in food that can act as antioxidants: vitamins C and E, carotenoids, selenium, manganese, glutathione, CoQ10, flavonoids, polyphenols, and the list goes on and on … And we are still finding more. Yes, supplementing with specific antioxidants might be helpful for unique health concerns, but don't count on them being a panacea. In fact, randomized placebo-controlled trials have shown that single antioxidant supplementation does not prevent cancer, heart disease, and other chronic conditions.[78]

Bottom line, as per usual, talk to your health-care provider to see if specific antioxidant support is necessary for you, and please: eat your veggies.

Fish Oil

This is a very common supplement for people to take. The benefits of having enough omega-3 fatty acids in your diet are many: better heart health, strong gut health, increased brain function, decreased inflammation, smoother skin, and on and on.[79] Historically, humans have had a really good balance of omega-6 to omega-3s from the foods we eat. As we have started replacing our healthy fatty food sources with processed fats and oils, this ratio has been thrown way off. For this reason, supplementing with fish oils has become more and more commonplace.[80]

Just like some amino acids, minerals, and vitamins, omega-3 fatty acids cannot be made within our bodies, so we have to get them from food. The best way to do this, of course, is by eating oily fish like mackerel, trout, and salmon. You can also get a good hit from shellfish (ahem ... just another reason I love oysters!).[81] Anyway, if you are not a fan of fish or can't eat it twice per week, then you might consider getting yourself a good fish oil supplement. Note, if you are eating grass-fed and pastured meats and dairy, you may already be getting a good amount of omega-3s from these meat sources. However, this applies *only* to grass-fed and finished and pasture-raised animals.[82] For you vegans out there, the only really good source of omega-3s will be sea vegetables like seaweed, chlorella, and spirulina. While some plant foods like chia seeds and flax have omega-3s in them, they are mainly in the form of ALA. This is a precursor to the DHA and EPA our bodies need, and the conversion rate is really low! Do not rely on seeds and nuts alone for their omega-3s.[83]

My biggest concern when it comes to recommending fish oil is quality. Please, oh please, do not purchase your fish oil in the bulk vitamin aisle at Costco. *Not only will a low-quality fish oil supplement not benefit you, but it can actually do more harm than good.* These oils are delicate and quickly oxidize (remember that word?) when subjected to heat and light. Avoid anything that is in a see-through bottle. As far as what to look for on the label, you want only the triglyceride forms of EPA and DHA on your labels. It should be clearly labeled where the fish comes from and which species. If not, there are likely multiple species from all over the world potentially mushed into your pills. That increases the time and processing, which translates to rancid fish oils by the time they end up in your shopping cart. Personally, I would refrigerate your fish oils (not in the door, but in the back of the fridge).[84]

Probiotics and Prebiotics

The bacteria that live in your gut really dictate how healthy your entire immune system is. We've already discussed the importance of gut health in the "Explore" chapter. We can keep those gut bugs happy and healthy by constantly repopulating them with varied species and feeding them the foods they need to proliferate. Probiotics are strains of bacteria that populate the gut making up your microbiota. Prebiotics are basically fertilizer that stimulates the growth of good bacteria in the gut. We actually need both of these to continuously aid our microbiota in being robust and staying healthy.[85]

I'm sure you'll be shocked to hear me say that you should first aim to get your prebiotics and probiotics from food. Probiotics will be found in any food that has undergone natural fermentation. The bacteria in these foods will resist our digestion, and those little bugs will then take root in our small intestines. Probiotic foods include things like yogurt, sauerkraut and kimchi, pickles, kefir, kombucha, sourdough, tempeh, miso, and soft cheeses. Prebiotics, on the other hand, are plant foods that are also resistant to our digestive system and instead are gobbled up by our gut bugs. You can feed your microbiome by consuming underripe bananas and plantains, dark chocolate (yes, for real), legumes, onions, garlic, leeks, Jerusalem artichokes, blueberries, spinach, dandelion greens, apples, oats, chia, and flax seeds.[86]

While you should really try to get a fair amount of both

probiotic and prebiotic foods in your diet to keep your gut healthy, there can be times when you might need a bit of a boost in the way of supplements. If you have been prescribed antibiotics lately, you might consider replenishing your gut bugs. Those antibiotics, regardless of the infection they are targeting, are indiscriminate in their attack of all bugs—good and bad.[87] Many of my clients who end up with a prescription for antibiotics have ensuing diarrhea, and I have found that when they pair their prescription with a good probiotic and prebiotic regimen, they feel much better. Of course, please defer to your prescribing doctor's advice before doing so.

Melatonin

This too is a rather controversial topic in the functional health realm. Some say it is a cure-all; others think you shouldn't touch the stuff. My take is somewhere in the middle. First of all, you should understand that melatonin is actually a hormone, not a vitamin or mineral.[88] This hormone is produced by your pineal gland and is said to be "a chemical expression of darkness." When your eyes perceive that light is changing and becoming more amber, then dark, the pineal gland starts to pump out melatonin. As melatonin levels rise, our need to sleep takes over. Levels of this sleep hormone seem to peak around 2 a.m. for most people. By the time we wake, it is back down to a low level.[89]

As we age, melatonin production decreases greatly. In

fact, by age fifty or sixty, many people barely make any at all. This is likely due to our decreased need for restorative sleep for growth and learning.[90] Like most hormones, if you supplement with it regularly, your body will not produce as much on its own. If you decide to take melatonin to help you reset your sleep pattern after suffering from jet lag, please take a low dose, and stop taking it when you feel your sleep is getting back on track.[91] I keep a melatonin spray in my nightstand drawer with a dose of 0.5 mg. When life stress is keeping me up, or I feel wired, a little spray under the tongue often does the trick. Sometimes I use only half a spray, which is 0.25 mg. Compare this to what many of my clients have told me they have taken: 5–10 mg and more! These are supra-physiological doses that far exceed anything your body would ever make on its own. These will not only knock you out but will also leave you feeling groggy in the morning.

While most of us think of melatonin as a chemical related to sleep, it is also a powerful anti-inflammatory.[92] Remember earlier when we learned about free radicals and how antioxidants combat them? Well, it turns out melatonin works in many areas of our bodies to scavenge those free radicals too. It's well shown now that melatonin can stop tissues from being damaged during inflammatory reactions. Since we tend to have an increase in inflammatory diseases as we get older, coupled with a natural decrease in melatonin, supplementation may actually be even more beneficial to those who are over the age of fifty.[93] Again, not at high doses, but a very low dose of melatonin if you have concerns about inflammation as you age might not be a bad idea. One word of caution: please check with your doctor if you are taking any other prescription medications, as melatonin seems to have adverse interactions with many drugs, including (but not limited to) birth control pills, fluvoxamine, warfarin, and immunosuppressants.[94]

And the List Goes On and On ...

Undoubtedly, some of you will have questions about some tincture or wonder potion that I haven't mentioned above. Things like turmeric, quercetin, collagen, and so on may be of interest to you. *Using the framework I have laid out for you at the end of this chapter, do your own research into individual supplements.* Also, consider what foods or other nutrients work with it synergistically, if you can get it from food sources, if there are toxicity concerns, and so on. Finally, ask yourself what you hope to get from taking said

Using the framework I have laid out for you at the end of this chapter, do your own research into individual supplements.

supplement. You can use websites like examine.com or labdoor.com to help you in your analysis. As always, please consult with your personal health-care practitioner to find the correct balance of supplementation. Lastly, once you decide to add new supplements into your health regimen, make a titration chart for yourself as we discussed earlier in this chapter. Always start with just one supplement at the lowest dose for a few days before slowly increasing up to the highest dose for your unique needs. Never forget your "why"!

Enhance Options

Supplement	What It Does (Why)	How Best to Take It	Who Should Consider It?	Is It Right for Me?
Vitamin C	Needed for immunity, strong bones and connective tissue, fights free radicals	Any time	Those with compromised immune systems, exposure to oxidative stress (smoking, inflammation), and if not eating plentiful fruits and veggies.	
B Complex	Getting energy from the food you eat, brain health, circulation, immunity, and detoxification	Any time, though some may find it energizing and should take in the morning.	Vegans, vegetarians, the elderly, and those with compromised digestion, mothers-to-be	
Vitamin A	Eye, reproduction, mucous membrane, and skin health	In combination with other fat-soluble vitamins, with food.	Vegans, and those with issues digesting fats	
Vitamin D	Bone strength, hormone production, immune system regulation	In combination with other fat-soluble vitamins, with food, and later in the day.	Low-fat dieters, those with dark complexions or who avoid the sun, the obese, and the elderly	
Vitamin E	Antioxidant, anticoagulant, immune boosting	With other fat-soluble vitamins, with a meal.	Low-fat dieters, those who don't digest fats well	
Vitamin K (1&2)	Bone health, circulation, calcium metabolism	In combination with other fat-soluble vitamins, with food.	Most people, especially those with concerns regarding calcium metabolism (low bone-density and heart disease). Anyone on statins and/or blood-thinning medications.	
Calcium	Bone health, muscle contraction (and heart health), nerve function, blood clotting	In combination with other fat-soluble vitamins, minerals, and with food. Take with vitamin K2, D3, Mg, etc.	Those with bone-density concerns, anyone who doesn't digest fats well, those who have taken corticosteroids, chemotherapy, or PPIs	
Magnesium	Blood pressure, mood, sleep, cardiovascular health, bone health, etc.	In the evenings generally, and with food. Take the version that is best for your needs.	Most people, those with sleep or mood disturbances, anyone with constipation	
Electrolytes	Proper hydration/fluid balance, muscle contraction	One coarse grain of quality sea salt per 16 oz. of filtered water.	Any time, especially with hard water, when exerting yourself, and with heat exposure	
Fish Oil	Decrease inflammation, support health of the gut, heart, brain, joints, etc.	With food	Anyone not consuming 2 servings of fish per week	
Probiotics and Prebiotics	Populate and feed healthy gut bugs	On an empty stomach	If having digestive health issues, not consuming probiotic and prebiotic foods, and when on an antibiotic course	
Melatonin	Normalizing circadian rhythm, anti-inflammatory	One hour before bed at the lowest possible dose	Anyone with sleep cycle issues, when jet-lagged, and anyone over the age of 50	

CHAPTER FIVE

Putting It All Together

Now it's time to finally put this whole wellness journey into actionable plans. Whether you skimmed through the various chapters, bounced back and forth, or read the whole thing straight through, you now know how to put all this information into the context of *you*. ***In these sections, you will distill all the workbook notes and put them into one cohesive action plan.*** You can find PDF copies of these at dfitlife. com/own-your-wellness-resources. Remember, the only constant is change, so when this new plan to "own your wellness" no longer suits you, come back and redo each section to course correct.

Before we whittle this down, I invite you to take a moment in self-reflection. I know you're eager to put all the new plans into place. But if you have made it this far, I know you are in it to win it. There's just one more piece of the puzzle that I think will take you even further in your journey.

In these sections, you will distill all the workbook notes and put them into one cohesive action plan.

Having a Vision

I have a few strategies I've picked up along the way that are helping me to keep evolving thoughtfully and purposefully.

I'm a huge believer in having a clear vision of your future. I used to use vision boards and make collages—and all that stuff is fun when you have the interest in hanging out at the craft store and making these goodies. The problem was that I really didn't like others seeing my vision board, and ideally, I'd like to have it in plain sight for myself. If I do not see it every day, it will not work. The other issue is that I like to morph these ideals as I see fit, and getting out the cardstock and coloring pencils every time just seemed a bit silly to me by the time I was in my forties.

Instead, here's what I do *every* day:

First of all, I set my alarm for about five minutes before I need to get moving. After I find my way to consciousness, and *before* I even look at my phone, I start my visions. For me, I have to close my eyes so I can really feel the visions, not just think of them. I believe that if I can really put myself (or whomever) into the picture, make it believable, and really know that it can happen, it has so much more power over me. I start going through each thing that really matters to me at the time and see how I want it to evolve.

This sounds oblique, I know, but here are the things that I envision at the time of writing this chapter. I'll even lay it out in the order I see it:

- I see my body lying in bed, lean and strong. I picture the strength of my bones—the whole skeleton, with attention to the strength of my leg bones, hip bones, vertebrae, and arms.

- Then I shift my attention to my husband lying next to me, not snoring (hee, hee), no belly fat from working long stressful days, his torso and arms strong and muscled. Then I see him flitter his eyes open, smile, and wrap me in his embrace.

- I then start seeing our children: the middle one happy and with friends exploring her college campus; the eldest clean-cut, standing with pride at our doorstep as he comes for a visit with his little dog, his self-purchased vehicle parked on our curb; then finally, our youngest, at her very statuesque adult height, long curls pulled into a ponytail, heading out for a jog with friends as she waves to me from the sidewalk.

- That vision helps me then turn my reflection to our home. Having purchased this amazing property we currently rent, we have renovated it into a clean-lined Spanish-style haven. The expansive kitchen is just off a light-filled entry that has stairs up to our primary suite. Our giant upstairs suite overlooks the backyard, which has a separate structure. In between are terra-cotta tiling and Mexican elders in a pathway leading to my private training studio and office. One wall of which is a roll-up garage-like door for tons of fresh air to come through.

- Inside that office is a mostly bare wall with some shelves carrying several copies of this book right here. My logo and *Own Your Wellness* grace the front.

- Finally, I see my bank accounts. I actually envision each app as I see it on my phone with exact dollar amounts. I even picture my credit card apps and the balances they hold.

So, that was maybe a bit of TMI. But I want you to understand how specific each vision is. I can't tell you how many times I've had to either eliminate one of my items or completely revamp it because what I had envisioned has come to be a reality. Countless times! What is hard to explain in the written word is how much I really *feel* the above items. I am there! It is really happening. What then ensues is that, even subconsciously, I make decisions throughout the day that bring these visions to life. I know it. I live it. I breathe it. Then it happens! Like magic, I swear.

But do you also see how this is constantly informing my "why?" When these visions and a sense of purpose are so vivid and current, I always have a "why." I have many. I'll put that darn weight vest on when I work out. Why? Because I need strong bones. I will make sure to encourage my husband's training, let him air out his grievances after a long day, and make sure there are vegetables for him to eat at home. Why? Because his health and happiness are critical to me. I could go on and on. But each decision I make throughout the day is informed by this five-minute vision practice. And that's really all it takes—five minutes!

Take a moment now and list out several things that

you'd like to envision. Take your time with it, and go through all the various facets of your life: relationships and loved ones, health, wealth, home, work, and so on.

Your Vision

_____

_____

_____

_____

_____

_____

_____

_____

_____

_____

I know it seems like a lot to "see," but the visions take only a few minutes. I really like lying in bed in the morning and starting my day with these visions. But you could schedule them into your day anywhere it seems ideal. Maybe you could make it part of a daily meditation or do it on your train commute to work. Maybe it happens while you're in the shower every day. What matters is that you do it often (ideally daily) to keep those priorities always informing your decisions. In the beginning, I used to have a list in the "notes" section of my smartphone to refer to, and I would think about my visions on my daily dog walk. You might want to print out your list and put it in your bathroom or office to see throughout the day. Try different ways, but make it happen. *You can manifest your ideal life (including your wellness) if the intention is there!* Full disclosure, I adapted this morning ritual after reading *Think and Grow Rich* by Napoleon Hill. It's some old-school thinking that leads to serious propulsion into building the life you have always aspired to. If you've never heard of this book, I highly recommend you give it a read. In the book *The Source* by Tara Swart MD, PhD, you can learn about the actual science behind how this works in your brain.

> You can manifest your ideal life (including your wellness) if the intention is there!

I've gotten pretty good about getting through my morning visions, so I've also added one more thing to the routine: "The One Thing." This isn't my original idea either.

I adopted this practice after reading the book *The One Thing* by Gary Keller and Jay Papasan. The general idea is to figure out the one thing I can do today to help propel myself closer to my goal. Then, what is the one thing I can do this week? This month? This year? So I do that in my head after I finish my envisioning. These change pretty often, especially the one thing of today and this week. But sometimes, even in the months and years, things evolve quicker than I mean them to. These ideas are critical as I navigate my choices, push through "to-do" lists, and constantly reevaluate where I'm setting my sights next.

Here's an example of what my "one thing" items are as of this morning:

- The one thing I need to do today: give my husband undivided attention and spend time to make sure he has a spectacular birthday.

- The one thing I need to do this week: get a good grasp of my income and expenditures this quarter as I plan out the impending holidays.

- The one thing I need to do this month: find a regular hitting partner so I can practice my tennis more regularly and make it fun.

- The one thing I need to do this year: find additional income streams to help move me closer to doubling my current income.

Ironically, the line, "The one thing I need to do …" has actually helped me move away from to-do lists per se and focus more on the larger concept of where I am going. Knowing what the end goal is but also being able to feel it, see it, and be in it makes it so much easier to focus my energies toward activities and projects that will help me achieve it. Instead of getting lost in the minutiae of little to-do lists, I can stay focused on what really matters! I encourage you to take a quick minute each day to work on figuring out your "one thing." You'll be surprised how much more effective your efforts feel.

I realize that it seems I've drifted more into the life-coaching side of things here, but of course, it is all connected. Whether you apply the above concepts to your fitness, stress management, career trajectory, relationship health, or finances, the same ideas apply:

Set a goal.

Know why you want to get there.

Streamline your efforts to get there as efficiently as possible.

Have fun along the way.

Your Goal, Your "Why," and Your Vision

We dove deep into the idea of fine-tuning not only your goal but why you want to achieve it and how it will *feel* when you do. Once you complete this section below, please put it up somewhere you can see it often. Maybe put copies in multiple places: inside your medicine cabinet, on the fridge, in your closet, wherever. *As you work through the action plan we will line up below, this will be your anchor.* Never lose sight of what the goal is, why you are reaching for it, and how it will feel to be there.

As you work through the action plan we will line up below, this will be your anchor.

My Goal(s)	Refer to page 20.
My Why	
My Vision	Go back to page 307 where you outlined how reaching this goal will feel for you, and put the main points here.

Nourish

In the first chapter, "Nourish," we spent a lot of time dialing in on your goals and being very specific with them. Hopefully, you already took the time to work through that section, but if

I wouldn't give yourself more than three things to work on here.

not, please flip back to the charts on pages 74, 77, 106, and 122. Here you should have already delineated some action items related to nourishing yourself. Below you will narrow them down to the most critical items needed to reach your goals. *I wouldn't give yourself more than three things to work on here.* The key is to keep it simple and not get overwhelmed.

Using those charts, here's an example for you to follow:

- Goal: Improve muscle tone by losing five inches around my waist.

- Why: Decrease my risk for heart disease and diabetes.

- Vision: Feel fit, have a good libido, enjoy time being active with my loved ones.

Action Items:

1. Wait until I'm hungry for breakfast.
2. Eat starches only at dinner.
3. Avoid snacks and eat plenty of protein with each meal.

Now, clearly, the action items I have set for the example goal do not exhaust all the options I could have implemented. There's no reason to. ***Start simple. Set yourself up for success.*** Once you conquer these, you can always go back and set up new plans to fine-tune how your nourishment will support your path to own your wellness.

Start simple. Set yourself up for success.

Goal	
Why	
Vision	
Action Item 1	
Action Item 2	
Action Item 3	

Move

Now, let's go back to the "Move" chapter and just tighten up what you put together. On page 128, you wrote out what movement practices you are doing day by day. Then on page 167, we got into great detail about each key element of movement and how you might incorporate them into your weekly routine. As a reminder, they include getting your heart rate up, getting and staying strong, keeping your balance, not getting too tight, and rest and recover.

Again, based on your goal(s) and "why," please line up for yourself which key elements you'll be incorporating day by day now. Remember, some of the real magic happens in the resting phase, so don't forget to give yourself a day or two in between those harder workouts. This can be fluid; feel free to come back and tweak this all you want. Try one version of it for a few weeks, then make adjustments. ***Keep your program evolving, and so will your physique!***

> **Keep your program evolving, and so will your physique!**

PUTTING IT ALL TOGETHER

Day of the Week	Movement Focus (Cardio, Strength, Balance, Stretching, or Rest)	Details (Length, Reps, Sets, Muscle Focus, Etc.)	Why (How It Supports Your Goal)
Monday			
Tuesday			
Wednesday			
Thursday			
Friday			
Saturday			
Sunday			

Explore

Once we lined up how best to nourish yourself and how to move, we dug deeper into the root causes of your symptoms. On page 197, you delineated your signs and symptoms of what is going on. Then, on page 202, you got a chance to riff on your origin story of where these issues may have started. You even worked on some sleuthing on page 205. Here you looked at each area of concern and found data points to start tracking. Lastly, we dove deep into some testing options for you, and you made some notes on the ones you might consider on page 253. We learned it's best to "test, not guess," because there's no point in throwing darts at some random target. *We want to zero in on the problem to efficiently and effectively devise a plan to get you feeling your best!*

Now we will take all of that and put it into one cohesive plan. This chart might take you a little longer than the Nourish and Move ones, but don't let that stop you. Go back to those other pages mentioned above and take the important bits from each. Once you're done with this, please find a health practitioner to help you with ordering any needed tests and interpreting them.

PUTTING IT ALL TOGETHER

Sign/Symptom	Possible Why	Data to Track	Testing to Consider
Poop			
Skin			
Sweat			
Aches/Pains			
Hunger/Cravings			
Sleep			
Mood			
Cognition			
Libido			

317

Enhance

Finally, we get to sprinkle on the supplements to enhance your wellness journey. Obviously, if you are working with a practitioner to do testing (as discussed above), they will likely make adjustments to the supplements you have determined you should take. But for now, go back to review the individual supplement chart on page 301. Whichever ones you decided might be helpful for you, use the titration chart on the next page to get started on your new regimen. Number one should be the supplement you feel is the most likely to positively impact your health. Then work down from there. Again, if this seems daunting, please reach out to your health practitioner for additional advice.

Titration Chart

Start with the lowest dose and increase slowly every
two to three days until you reach the maximum dosage.
Do not go to the next supplement without
completing titration of previous.

Supplement by Priority	Starting Dose	Maximal Dose	Timing/ Instructions	Reason for Taking	Notes
1.					
2.					
3.					
4.					
5.					
6.					

Thank You

THANK YOU

I want to thank you for taking the time to go on this journey with me. Owning your wellness is not easy. Heck, owning up to anything in your life takes courage. Being honest with yourself about why you need to work on certain areas of your life is a seriously hard thing to do. It's much easier to just put the onus on someone or something else. You could simply blame your circumstances. Life often just deals us a crappy hand. *But by reading this book, you have decided to not play the victim in the story of your life, but to be the protagonist! You are owning your wellness.*

By walking you through this process, it has allowed me to own my personal wellness too. Not only in the literal sense that each chapter I wrote forced me to sit down and really think about the adjustments I had to make to my own Nourish, Move, Explore, and Enhance areas of life, but in the macro sense of sharing my process. I hope that you will be able now to use this formula to continually move forward, course correct, and reach ever-growing

By reading this book, you have decided to not play the victim in the story of your life, but to be the protagonist! You are owning your wellness.

heights of wellness. I hope you will share this process with friends, family, and anyone who needs guidance. And who doesn't?

In the last year of writing this, I had to make some serious changes to my own wellness journey. Even though my goal (attaining and maintaining strong bones) and my "why" (to live a long, highly active, and healthy life) have not changed, the how sure has.

Nourish: I am currently back to daily fasts of fourteen to fifteen hours to help with detoxification and metabolic health. I am eating a high-fat diet of 55 percent most days of the week. And I'm making sure to get at least one higher carb and higher calorie refeed weekly or biweekly.

Move: I have started getting back to really, really heavy lifting once or twice a week to get those bones super strong. I'm doing more yoga to keep myself supple and to help with stress management. Finally, I'm trying to get my dog out for longer walks daily so we both get a good dose of vitamin D and feel-good endorphins.

Explore: I realized that maybe the occasional bloating and gas I'm experiencing is actually an issue, so I will be ordering the GI-MAP for myself. I have also taken the Metabolic Typing Diet questionnaire to validate that I'm a fast oxidizer and need lots of fat and protein to function at my best. I continue to order the DUTCH and thyroid labs for myself at least twice per year and review them with my doctor.

Enhance: This last year I have really dialed in the vitamins and minerals I need to maximize my bone health. I have also come up with a pretty good cocktail of magnesium, vitamin D, and phosphatidylserine to help me drift off to sleep better.

You are not in this alone! Aside from this book, you can find me online in various ways. There are many people going through similar issues right now. Together, we can go far! Please go to my website, dfitlife.com, for the latest information on how to contact me and how to join my online community to keep learning how to own your wellness.

From the bottom of my heart, thank you.

Yours in health,
Daniella

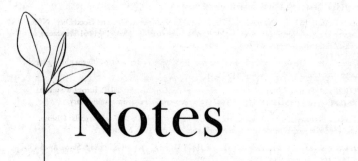

Notes

1. Julia Reedy, How the U.S. Low-Fat Diet Recommendations of 1977 Contributed to the Declining Health of Americans, April 29, 2016, https://digitalcommons.lib.uconn.edu/cgi/viewcontent.cgi?article=1482&context=srhonors_theses.

2. "History of USDA Nutrition Guidelines," Wikipedia, December 6, 2023, https://en.wikipedia.org/wiki/History_of_USDA_nutrition_guidelines.

3. Maria Godoy, "Wheels, Pyramids and Plates: USDA's Struggles to Illustrate Good Diet," NPR, January 13, 2016, https://www.npr.org/sections/thesalt/2016/01/13/462821161/illustrating-diet-advice-is-hard-heres-how-usda-has-tried-to-do-it.

4. Walter Willett, "Reassessing the Food Pyramid," PBS, April 8, 2004, https://www.pbs.org/wgbh/pages/frontline/shows/diet/themes/pyramid.html.

5. "USDA's MyPlate Celebrates Its First Anniversary," USDA, May 30, 2012, https://www.usda.gov/media/press-releases/2012/05/30/usdas-myplate-celebrates-its-first-anniversary.

6. Ghada A. Soliman, Dietary Cholesterol and the Lack of Evidence in Cardiovascular Disease, June 16, 2018, https://www.ncbi.nlm.nih.gov/pmc/articles/PMC6024687/.

7. Shawn Stevenson, "The 13 Rules Of Health That I Live By," The Model Health Show, April 15, 2019, https://themodelhealthshow.com/13-rules-of-health-that-i-live-by/.

8. "Avocados," The Nutrition Source, February 2, 2023, https://www.hsph.harvard.edu/nutritionsource/avocados/#:~:text=Did%20You%20Know.

9. Matthew M. Schubert et al., Impact of 4 Weeks of Interval Training on Resting Metabolic Rate, Fitness, and Health-Related Outcomes, October 24, 2017, https://pubmed.ncbi.nlm.nih.gov/28633001/.

10. Bari Lieberman, How Long Should You Rest Between Intervals?, March 31, 2014, https://www.prevention.com/fitness/fitness-tips/a20470388/the-optimal-amount-of-time-to-rest-between-intervals/.

11. Sigrid Breit et al., Vagus Nerve as Modulator of the Brain–Gut Axis in Psychiatric and Inflammatory Disorders, March 13, 2018, https://www.ncbi.nlm.nih.gov/pmc/articles/PMC5859128/#:~:text=The%20vagus%20nerve.

12. Hormonal Acne: What Is It, Treatment, Causes & Prevention, accessed December 7, 2023, https://my.clevelandclinic.org/health/diseases/21792-hormonal-acne.

13. Ronald Prussick, Lisa Prussick, and Dillon Nussbaum, "Nonalcoholic Fatty Liver Disease and Psoriasis," U.S. National Library of Medicine, March 2015, https://www.ncbi.nlm.nih.gov/pmc/articles/PMC4382145/.

14. Hypohidrosis: Symptoms, Causes, Complications, and More, accessed December 7, 2023, https://www.webmd.com/skin-problems-and-treatments/what-is-hypohidrosis.

15. Reference Ranges and What They Mean, July 9, 2021, https://www.testing.com/articles/laboratory-test-reference-ranges/#:~:text=Individual.

16. "Diabetes Tests," Centers for Disease Control and Prevention, February 28, 2023, https://www.cdc.gov/diabetes/basics/getting-tested.html#:~:text=Fasting%20Blood%20Sugar.

17. "All about Your A1c," Centers for Disease Control and Prevention, September 30, 2022, https://www.cdc.gov/diabetes/managing/managing-blood-sugar/a1c.html; Xiaohong Zhang et al., Fasting Insulin, Insulin Resistance, and Risk of Cardiovascular or All-Cause Mortality in Non-Diabetic Adults: A Meta-Analysis, September 7, 2017, https://www.ncbi.nlm.nih.gov/pmc/articles/PMC6448479/.

18. William C. Cromwell and Thomas A. Barringer, Low-density lipoprotein and Apolipoprotein B: Clinical use in patients with coronary heart disease, November 11, 2009, https://pubmed.ncbi.nlm.nih.gov/19863872/.

19. Michael Ruscio, "What Are Optimal Thyroid Levels?," Dr. Michael Ruscio, DC, September 5, 2020, https://drruscio.com/optimal-thyroid-levels/.

20. Eve Henry, "A Functional Medicine Approach to Thyroid Hormone Labs," Rupa Health, March 3, 2023, https://www.rupahealth.com/post/a-functional-medicine-approach-to-thyroid-hormone-labs#:~:text=The%20typical%20reference%20range%20provided,appropriate%20for%20most%20healthy%20adults.

21. "Hypoglycemia," Mayo Clinic, November 18, 2023, https://www.mayoclinic.org/diseases-conditions/hypoglycemia/symptoms-causes/syc-20373685#:~:text=Hypoglycemia%20needs%20immediate%20treatment.

22. Michael Roussell and Thu Huynh, "What Is Postprandial Blood Sugar and Why Does It Matter?," Levels, October 12, 2023, https://www.levelshealth.com/blog/what-is-postprandial-blood-sugar-and-why-does-it-matter.

23. Daniella Dayoub Forrest, "Want to Optimize Your Health? Check Your Thyroid First!," DFitLife, October 12, 2020, https://www.dfitlife.com/post/want-to-optimize-your-health-check-your-thyroid-first.

24. "Thyroid Hormone: What It Is & Function," Cleveland Clinic, accessed December 7, 2023, https://my.clevelandclinic.org/health/articles/22391-thyroid-hormone.

25. Todd B. Nippoldt, "Thyroid Peroxidase Antibody Test: What Is It?," Mayo Clinic, July 16, 2022, https://www.mayoclinic.org/thyroid-disease/expert-answers/faq-20058114#:~:text=TPO%20plays%20an%20important%20role,to%20help%20find%20the%20cause.

26. "Hypothyroidism (Underactive Thyroid)," Mayo Clinic, December 10, 2022, https://www.mayoclinic.org/diseases-conditions/hypothyroidism/symptoms-causes/syc-20350284#:~:text=The%20most%20common%20cause%20of,process%20involves%20320%20Note%20s%20%20your%20thyroid%20gland.

27. Melinda Smith, "Vitamins and Minerals," HelpGuide.org, February 24, 2023, https://www.helpguide.org/harvard/vitamins-and-minerals.htm.

28. "Vitamin C," Mayo Clinic, August 10, 2023, https://www.mayoclinic.org/drugs-supplements-vitamin-c/art-20363932.

29. "Foods High in B Vitamins," WebMD, accessed December 7, 2023, https://www.webmd.com/diet/foods-high-in-b-vitamins#1.

30. Stephanie Eckelkamp, "What Exactly Is Methylation & Why Is It So Essential to Overall Health?," mindbodygreen, accessed December 7, 2023, https://www.mindbodygreen.com/articles/what-is-methylation.

31. Jillian Kubala, "B-Complex Vitamins: Benefits, Side Effects, and Dosage," Healthline, April 21, 2023, https://www.healthline.com/nutrition/vitamin-b-complex#overview.

32. Fat-Soluble Vitamins, accessed December 7, 2023, https://www.ncbi.nlm.nih.gov/books/NBK218749/.

33. "Vitamin A," Mayo Clinic, September 14, 2023, https://www.mayoclinic.org/drugs-supplements-vitamin-a/art-20365945.

34. "Vitamin D," The Nutrition Source, March 7, 2023, https://www.hsph.harvard.edu/nutritionsource/vitamin-d/#:~:text=It%20is%20a%20fat%2Dsolu-ble.

35. Megan Ware, "Vitamin D: Benefits, Deficiency, Sources, and Dosage," Medical News Today, accessed December 7, 2023, https://www.medicalnewstoday.com/articles/161618.

36. "25-Hydroxy Vitamin D Test," Mount Sinai Health System, accessed December 7, 2023, https://www.mountsinai.org/health-library/tests/25-hydroxy-vitamin-d-test#:~:text=The%20nor-mal%20range%20of%20vitamin.

37. "Vitamin E," The Nutrition Source, March 7, 2023, https://www.hsph.harvard.edu/nutritionsource/vitamin-e/#:~:text=Vitamin%20E%20is%20a%20.

38. Chris Kresser, "Vitamin K2: The Missing Nutrient," Chris Kresser, August 25, 2023,

https://chriskresser.com/vitamin-k2-the-missing-nutrient/.

39. Katarzyna Maresz, "Proper Calcium Use: Vitamin K2 as a Promoter of Bone and Cardiovascular Health," Integrative medicine (Encinitas, Calif.), February 2015, https://www.ncbi.nlm.nih.gov /pmc/articles/PMC4566462/.

40. "Vitamin K," NIH Office of Dietary Supplements, accessed December 7, 2023, https://ods.od .nih.gov/factsheets/VitaminK-HealthProfessional/.

41. Toshiro Sato, Naoko Inaba, and Takatoshi Yamashita, MK-7 and Its Effects on Bone Quality and Strength, March 31, 2020, https://www.ncbi.nlm.nih.gov/pmc/articles/PMC7230802/; Mark Sisson, "Dear Mark: What Are the Differences between Vitamin K2 Mk-4 and Mk-7?," Mark's Daily Apple, September 19, 2019, https://www.marksdailyapple.com/what-are-the -differences-between-vitamin-k2-mk-4-and-mk-7/.

42. "Vitamins and Minerals," The Nutrition Source, March 8, 2023, https://www.hsph.harvard.edu /nutritionsource/vitamins/#:~:text=Vitamins%20and%20miner-als%20are%20micronutrients.

43. Karey Thomas, "Calcium, Your Diet, and the Cofactor Cycle," Dr. Drew Huffman, May 21, 2020, https://drdrewhuffman.com/2020/05/21/calcium-your-diet-and-the-cofactor-cycle/.

44. "Calcium," The Nutrition Source, March 7, 2023, https://www.hsph.harvard.edu/nutritionsource /calcium/#:~:text=Calcium%20is%20a%20mineral% 20most,heart%20rhythms%20and%20 nerve%20functions.

45. Kerri-Ann Jennings and Rachael Ajmera, "Top 15 Calcium-Rich Foods (Many Are Nondairy)," Healthline, August 2, 2023, https://www.healthline.com/nutrition/15-calcium-rich-foods#TOC _TITLE_HDR_5.

46. Thomas, "Calcium."

47. "Phosphorus," Mount Sinai Health System, accessed December 7, 2023, https://www.mountsinai. org/health-library/supplement/phosphorus#:~:text=Phosphorus%20.

48. "Phosphorus and Your Diet," National Kidney Foundation, September 8, 2023, https://www .kidney.org/atoz/content/phosphorus#how-can-i-control-my-phosphorus-level.

49. "Phosphorus," The Nutrition Source, March 7, 2023, https://www.hsph.harvard.edu/nutrition source/phosphorus/.

50. "Chloride in Diet," Mount Sinai Health System, accessed December 8, 2023, https://www. mountsinai.org/health-library/nutrition/chloride-in-diet#:~:text=Function,of%20%20digestive%20 (stomach)%20juices.

51. "Office of Dietary Supplements - Magnesium," NIH Office of Dietary Supplements, accessed December 8, 2023, https://ods.od.nih.gov/factsheets/Magnesium-Consumer/.

52. R. Swaminathan, Magnesium Metabolism and Its Disorders, May 2003, https://www.ncbi.nlm .nih.gov/pmc/articles/PMC1855626/.

53. Korin Miller, "Nine Different Types of Magnesium + When You Need Each One," mindbody-green, accessed December 8, 2023, https://www.mindbodygreen.com/articles/magnesium -supplement-types; "Types of Magnesium," Balance Women's Health, accessed December 8, 2023, https://balance womenshealth.com/wp-content/uploads/2020/03/PE-H-Types-of-Magnesium.pdf.

54. "Potassium," The Nutrition Source, March 7, 2023, https://www.hsph.harvard.edu/nutritionsource/ potassium/#:~:text=Potassium%20is%20found%20 naturally%20in,and%20supports%20 normal%20blood%20pressure.

55. "Nutrition's Dynamic Duos," Harvard Health, July 1, 2009, https://www.health.harvard.edu /newsletter_article/Nutritions-dynamic-duos.

56. "Sodium, Potassium and Health," Centers for Disease Control and Prevention, August 23, 2022, https://www.cdc.gov/salt/potassium.htm.

57. "Ten Foods That Are High in Potassium," Cleveland Clinic, November 27, 2023,

NOTES

Notes

https://health.clevelandclinic.org/10-foods-that-are-high-in-potassium.

58. Laura Dan, "Sulfur Rich Foods: Benefits and Best Sources," Fullscript, October 19, 2023, https://fullscript.com/blog/sulfur-rich-foods.

59. "Electrolytes: Types, Purpose & Normal Levels," Cleveland Clinic, accessed December 8, 2023, https://my.clevelandclinic.org/health/diagnostics/21790-electrolytes.

60. "Fluid and Electrolyte Balance," U.S. National Library of Medicine, accessed December 8, 2023, https://medlineplus.gov/fluidandelectrolytebalance.html#:~:text=Sodium%2C.

61. Ashley Lall, "Make Your Own Electrolyte Water for Free with This Easy Hack," Woman's World, February 26, 2020, https://www.womansworld.com/posts/health/how-to-make-electrolyte-water.

62. "Eight Essential Trace Minerals Your Body Needs - Are You Getting Enough?," Brain Balance, accessed December 8, 2023, https://www.brainbalancecenters.com/blog/trace-minerals-important-health; Diet and Health: Implications for Reducing Chronic Disease Risk, accessed December 8, 2023, https://www.ncbi.nlm.nih.gov/books/NBK218751/.

63. Rhonda Anderson-Lauritzen, "Trace Mineral Deficiency," Mineral Resources International Inc., March 31, 2023, https://www.mineralresourcesint.com/trace-mineral-deficiency-9-facts-you-need-to-know-2/#:~:text=Trace%20minerals%20serve%20many%20functions.

64. Rachel Mantock, "We Need to Talk about IUDs and Copper Toxicity," The Femedic, September 9, 2019, https://thefemedic.com/contraception/we-need-to-talk-about-iuds-and-copper-toxicity/.

65. Yvette Brazier, "Why Do We Have Fluoride in Our Water?," Medical News Today, February 21, 2018, https://www.medicalnewstoday.com/articles/154164.

66. "Iodine Deficiency," American Thyroid Association, accessed December 8, 2023, https://www.thyroid.org/iodine-deficiency/#:~:text=Iodine%20is%20an%20element%20that.

67. "Iron Deficiency Anemia," Mayo Clinic, accessed December 8, 2023, https://www.mayoclinic.org/diseases-conditions/iron-deficiency-anemia/symptoms-causes/syc-20355034.

68. "Iron," The Nutrition Source, March 7, 2023, https://www.hsph.harvard.edu/nutritionsource/iron/#:~:text=Heme%20is%20found%20only.

69. "Manganese," Mount Sinai Health System, accessed December 8, 2023, https://www.mountsinai.org/health-library/supplement/manganese#:~:text=Manganese%20.

70. "Molybdenum," NIH Office of Dietary Supplements, accessed December 8, 2023, https://ods.od.nih.gov/factsheets/Molybdenum-Consumer/.

71. Henry A. Spiller, "Rethinking Mercury: The Role of Selenium in the Pathophysiology of Mercury Toxicity," U.S. National Library of Medicine, May 2018, https://pubmed.ncbi.nlm.nih.gov/29124976/#:~:text=Selenium%20supplementation%20has.

72. "Selenium," NIH Office of Dietary Supplements, accessed December 8, 2023, https://ods.od.nih.gov/factsheets/Selenium-HealthProfessional/.

73. A. S. Prasad et al., "Zinc Status and Serum Testosterone Levels of Healthy Adults," U.S. National Library of Medicine, May 1996, https://pubmed.ncbi.nlm.nih.gov/8875519/.

74. "Foods High in Zinc and Why You Need It," WebMD, accessed December 8, 2023, https://www.webmd.com/diet/foods-high-in-zinc#1.

75. Anne Marie Helmenstine, "Understand What Oxidation Means in Chemistry," ThoughtCo, February 12, 2020, https://www.thoughtco.com/definition-of-oxidation-in-chemistry-605456.

76. V. Lobo et al., "Free Radicals, Antioxidants and Functional Foods: Impact on Human Health," U.S. National Library of Medicine, July 2010, https://www.ncbi.nlm.nih.gov/pmc/articles/PMC3249911/.

77. "Antioxidant Supplements: What You Need to Know," U.S. Department of Health and Human Services, accessed December 8, 2023, https://www.nccih.nih.gov/health/antioxidant-supple

ments-what-you-need-to-know.

78. "Antioxidants," The Nutrition Source, March 3, 2021, https://www.hsph.harvard.edu/nutrition source/antioxidants/.

79. Ruairi Robertson, "12 Important Benefits of Fish Oil, Based on Science," Healthline, accessed December 8, 2023, https://www.healthline.com/nutrition/benefits-of-fish-oil.

80. Cynthia A. Daley et al., "A Review of Fatty Acid Profiles and Antioxidant Content in Grass-Fed and Grain-Fed Beef," Nutrition journal, March 10, 2010, https://www.ncbi.nlm.nih.gov/pmc /articles/PMC2846864/.

81. "Fish Oil," Mayo Clinic, August 10, 2023, https://www.mayoclinic.org/drugs-supplements -fish-oil/art-20364810.

82. Daley, "Review of Fatty Acid."

83. Kat Gál and Charlotte Lillis, "15 Foods That Are Very High in Omega-3," Medical News Today, accessed December 8, 2023, https://www.medicalnewstoday.com/articles/323144.

84. Lauren Del Turco, "Your Fish Oil Supplement Might Not Be as High-Quality as You Think," mindbodygreen, accessed December 8, 2023, https://www.mindbodygreen.com/articles/what -to-look-for-in-high-quality-fish-oil-supplement.

85. Gail Cresci, "Prebiotics vs. Probiotics: What's the Difference?," Cleveland Clinic, November 27, 2023, https://health.clevelandclinic.org/prebiotics-vs-probiotics-whats-the-difference/; Katherine Zeratsky, "Probiotics and Prebiotics: What You Should Know," Mayo Clinic, July 2, 2022, https:// www.mayoclinic.org/prebiotics-probiotics-and-your-health/art-20390058.

86. "Foods with Probiotics That Help Digestion," WebMD, accessed December 8, 2023, https://www.webmd.com/digestive-disorders/ss/slideshow-probiotics.

87. Blake Rodgers, Kate Kirley, and Anne Mounsey, "Prescribing an Antibiotic? Pair It with Probiotics," U.S. National Library of Medicine, March 2013, https://www.ncbi.nlm.nih.gov/pmc/articles /PMC3601687/.

88. "Melatonin," Mayo Clinic, August 10, 2023, https://www.mayoclinic.org/drugs-supplements -melatonin/art-20363071.

89. Theodoros B. Grivas and Olga D. Savvidou, "Melatonin the 'Light of Night' in Human Biology and Adolescent Idiopathic Scoliosis," U.S. National Library of Medicine, April 4, 2007, https://www.ncbi.nlm.nih.gov/pmc/articles/PMC1855314/#:~:text=Synthesis%20of %20 melatonin%2Dthe%20role,inhibited%20by%20light%20%5B4%5D.

90. Grivas, "Melatonin."

91. Brent A. Bauer, "Pros and Cons of Melatonin," Mayo Clinic, October 28, 2022, https://www.may- oclinic.org/healthy-lifestyle/adult-health/expert-answers/melatonin-side-effects /faq-20057874#:~ :text=Melatonin%20is%20generally%20safe%20for,Headache

92. Anna Tarocco et al., "Melatonin as a Master Regulator of Cell Death and Inflammation: Molecular Mechanisms and Clinical Implications for Newborn Care," Nature News, April 8, 2019, https:// www.nature.com/articles/s41419-019-1556-7#:~:text=Melatonin%20as%20a%20 potent%20 and%20widespread%20anti%2Dinflammatory%20agent&text=Experimental%20 and%20 clinical%20data%20suggest,various%20pathophysiological%20situations73%2C74.

93. R. J. Reiter et al., "Melatonin and Its Relation to the Immune System and Inflammation," U.S. National Library of Medicine, accessed December 8, 2023, https://pubmed.ncbi.nlm .nih.gov/11268363/; Joshua H. Cho et al., "Anti-Inflammatory Effects of Melatonin: A Systematic Review and Meta-Analysis of Clinical Trials," ScienceDirect, February 10, 2021, https://www.sciencedirect .com/science/article/abs/pii/S0889159121000386.

94. "Melatonin - Uses, Side Effects, and More," WebMD, accessed December 8, 2023, https://www.webmd.com/vitamins/ai/ingredientmono-940/melatonin.

If you want to continue learning how to
"Own your wellness,"
Please visit DFitLife.com

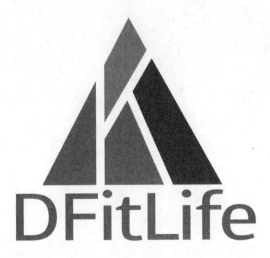

You will find links to sign up for Daniella's blog,
a self-paced course to further own your wellness
and access other learning resources.

If you'd like personal wellness coaching
one-on-one with Daniella, email her directly
at Daniella@DFitLife.com.

To download all the resources
within this book, please visit
www.dfitlife.com/own-your-wellness-resources